Court Battles over a Pollution-Related Disease
The Case of Minamata Disease

英語版・日本語版

ノーモア・ミナマタ
司法による解決のみち

水俣病不知火患者会
ノーモア・ミナマタ国賠等訴訟弁護団
ノーモア・ミナマタ編集委員会
【編】

【監訳】
鳥飼香代子
（南栄科技大学教授、前熊本大学教授）

土肥勲嗣
（九州大学大学院法学研究院専門研究員）

Edited by
Association of Minamata Disease Victims "SHIRANUI," No-More-Minamata Defense Team, and No-More-Minamata Editing Committee

Translation supervised by
Kayoko Torikai (Professor of Housing and Urban Planning at Nan Jeon University of Science and Technology, Taiwan, and former Professor at Kumamoto University, Japan) and
Kunji Doi (Research Fellow of the Faculty of Law at Kyushu University, Japan)

花伝社

目 次

英語版
Court Battles over a Pollution-Related Disease
The Case of Minamata Disease　　　　　　　　　　　i

日本語版
ノーモア・ミナマタ
司法による解決のみち　　　　　　　　　　　75

Court Battles
over
a Pollution-Related Disease
The Case of Minamata Disease

Edited by
Association of Minamata Disease Victims "SHIRANUI," No-More-Minamata Defense Team, and No-More-Minamata Editing Committee

Translation supervised by
Kayoko Torikai (Professor of Housing and Urban Planning at Nan Jeon University of Science and Technology, Taiwan, and former Professor at Kumamoto University, Japan) and
Kunji Doi (Research Fellow of the Faculty of Law at Kyushu University, Japan)

Members of the No-More-Minamata Editing Committee
   Kunji Doi 土肥勲嗣 (Research Fellow at Kyushu University)
   Takaaki Ikai 猪飼隆明 (Professor Emeritus at Osaka University)
   Masaru Itai 板井優 (Lawyer)
   Hideo Kitaoka 北岡秀郎 (Nonfiction writer)
   Toshio Oishi 大石利生 (Chair of the Association of Minamata Disease Victims "SHIRANUI")
   Syoto Sonoda 園田昭人 (Lawyer)
   Kayoko Torikai 鳥飼香代子 (Professor at Nan Jeon University of Science and Technology and former Professor at Kumamoto University)
   Shinji Tsubohara 坪原紳二 (Momoki Saito Architects)

   Chair and contact person: Takaaki Ikai
                  20-5 Kokubu 1-chome, Chuo-ku, Kumamoto-shi
                  Kumamoto 862-0949, Japan
                  Tel: 096-362-0570

Translated by Shinji Tsubohara

First published on October 1, 2013

All rights reserved. No part of this publication may be reproduced, stored in a retrieval system or transmitted in any form or by any means, electronic, mechanical, photocopying, recording or otherwise without the prior permission of the publisher.

Published by
Kadensha
Shuppan Yuso Building 2nd Floor
5-11 Nishikanda 2-chome, Chiyoda-ku
Tokyo 101-0065
Japan

Contents

List of Photos v
List of Figures v
Preface vi
Notes on the Contributors viii

Introduction: The Role of Justice in Modern Japanese Society 1
Takaaki Ikai

Chapter 1. The History of Minamata Disease 17

Chapter 2. The Record of Battle in the No-More-Minamata 35
Lawsuit Claiming Government Compensation

Chapter 3. The Content and Achievements of the 2011 61
Victorious Settlement

Conclusion: Remaining Minamata Disease Issues 71

Japanese Version 75

Appendices 129
Index 141

List of Photos

1. Minamata Bay before Chisso came	20
2. Minamata Bay before Chisso came	20
3. Meisuien, a special hospital for Minamata disease	22
4. Minamata disease victim	23
5. Polluter Chisso Minamata factory	27
6. First Kumamoto Minamata Disease Lawsuit	29
7. Third Kumamoto Minamata Disease Lawsuit	31
8. Minamata disease victim	37
9. Meeting of victims	41
10. Meeting of victims	42
11. Departure ceremony of the Minamata Caravan	54
12. Street campaign	55
13. General meeting of plaintiffs on March 21, 2011	65
14. Dumpsters for contaminated fish	72
15. Global interest in Minamata disease	72

List of Figures

1. Japan and the four big pollution trials	12
2. Chisso and Minamata City	18
3. Shiranui Sea	36
4. Employed persons by industry	137
5. Population change by age group	137

Preface

Minamata disease is extremely tragic and serious human damage caused by industrial activity. Therefore, it is called the starting point of pollution.

Minamata disease is a pollution-related disease: victims contracted it by eating large amounts of fish and shellfish contaminated with methyl mercury, which was contained in wastewater released from the Minamata factory of Chisso in Minamata City, Kumamoto Prefecture. It was officially recognized on May 1, 1956.

While recognizing the outbreak of Minamata disease, Chisso continued to discharge wastewater untreated into the Shiranui Sea. Although they could have prevented the outbreak and spread of the disease, the national and Kumamoto prefectural governments prioritized economic growth, neglecting to take appropriate preventive measures. As a result, many people contracted it.

Victims of Minamata disease present various symptoms ranging from serious human damage of dying in madness to a relatively mild symptom of sensory disorders alone. The clinical picture of the disease is not yet completely elucidated. In addition, when the contamination was serious, there were about 200,000 people living in the costal areas of the Shiranui Sea, many of whom surely ate large amounts of contaminated fish and shellfish. But the number of victims there is not revealed, because governments have neglected a comprehensive investigation.

Victims of Minamata disease have waged battles against the offending company and governments — who have denied damage — claiming compensation over more than half a century.

Even after the October 2004 Supreme Court decision in favor of victims and the enactment of the Law Concerning Special Measures for the Relief of Minamata Disease Victims and the Settlement of Minamata Disease Issues in July 2009, victims who do not yet receive compensation

Preface

continue their battle. On June 20, 2013, forty-eight victims whose applications for compensation based on the law had been rejected filed a new lawsuit. That is why the battle by victims is still underway.

Minamata disease issues have followed a highly complex and extraordinary course, because the offending company and governments have consistently failed to prevent pollution, conduct investigations, and acknowledge the seriousness of damage. Such mistakes must serve as a negative lesson in preventing pollution and compensating victims in other countries. It is fortunate if this book can contribute to that goal.

Syoto Sonoda
Lawyer

Notes on the Contributors

Takaaki Ikai is Professor Emeritus at Osaka University and a historian. He has studied political history, the history of ideas, and the history of social movements after the last days of the Tokugawa regime and the Meiji Restoration. His main works include *Takamori Saigo* (Iwanami Shinsho), *The Satsuma Rebellion: Justification for the War and the Mobilized People* (Yoshikawa Kobunkan), *Hannah Riddell and Kaishun Hospital* (Kumamoto Publishing Cultural Association), and *The Meiji Secret History of Kumamoto* (Kumamoto Nichinichi Shimbun). Concerning Minamata disease issues, among his publications are *Premises Underpinning Minamata Disease Issues* and *The Corporate Activities of Chisso Backed by National Policy*. He also served as the chair of the screening committee for the No-More-Minamata Environmental Award.

Hideo Kitaoka is a nonfiction writer. He was born in Kumamoto City in 1943. After working as high-school teacher, he had been a staff member of the defense team for Minamata disease lawsuits since 1971. From 1975 to 1996, he had published a monthly periodical, *Minamata*, bringing public attention to Minamata disease issues. He served as the secretary of the Kumamoto Prefecture Liaison Council to Support Minamata Disease Battles, the secretary of the National Liaison Council to Support Hansen's Disease Lawsuit Claiming Government Compensation, and the secretary of the Liaison Council to Support the Kawabe River Irrigation Lawsuit. Through publications, he continues to disseminate information about wide-ranging issues including Minamata disease, Hansen's disease, the Kawabe River Dam, lawsuits by atomic bomb survivors, and nuclear accidents.

Notes on the Contributors

Masaru Itai is a lawyer. He had been devoted to settling Minamata disease issues as the secretary of the defense team for Minamata disease lawsuits for eight years and six months, with his law office located in Minamata City. He helped substantially stop the Kawabe River Dam construction project, which could destroy the environment. He is the secretary of the Western Japan Defense Team for Hansen's Disease Lawsuit Claiming Government Compensation. Tackling pollution problems, he has consecutively been the secretary, executive head, and deputation of the National Liaison Council of Pollution Defense Teams. He is now engaged in a battle to decommission a nuclear power plant as the joint representative of the defense team for the "Eliminate the Nuclear Power Plant! Kyushu Genkai Lawsuit."

Introduction

The Role of Justice in Modern Japanese Society

Takaaki Ikai

This book aims to reveal the fact that a company's production activities backed by national policy inflicted extremely serious damage, "Minamata disease," on local residents and laborers, and describe an extensive and prolonged battle mainly on the judicial front to relieve the victims. To elucidate the meaning and significance of the battle centering on the judicial front, this chapter will present what kind of role justice played in modern Japanese society particularly after the Meiji Restoration, and how it has changed since after World War II.

1. The Judicial System before World War II

"*Seitaisho*" promulgated on intercalary fourth month twenty-first day, 1868, stipulated the separation of powers — executive, judiciary, and legislative — according to the modern legal system while it concentrated power on the Grand Council of State; it established courts of justice in Osaka, Hyogo, Nagasaki, Kyoto, Yokohama, and Hakodate. This was the beginning of the judicial system of modern Japan, but these courts were equivalent to local executive offices, not independent judicial offices. On July 9, 1871, immediately after the abolition of feudal domains and the establishment of prefectures, the Department of Justice was established, with the department's court, prefectural courts, and municipal courts introduced. These courts, however, still worked as local executive offices.

It was after the Supreme Court was established on April 1, 1875, and jurisdiction was transferred form the Minister of Justice to this court that the Japanese judicial system overcame such character, to a certain extent, and took the first step toward realizing the modern Japanese judicial system. Namely, this reform introduced a hierarchy from the Supreme Court to high courts (Tokyo, Osaka, Nagasaki, Fukushima, and, later, Miyagi) to prefectural courts (turned into district courts next year), enacting the Regulations as to Organizations of the Supreme Court and the Other Courts, the Proceedings of Intermediate and Final Appeals, and the Conduct of Judicial Proceedings.

Subsequently, to counter the growing Freedom and People's Rights Movement, the national government promulgated the Criminal Law and the Criminal Procedure Law on July 17, 1880. Adopting the principle of "nulla poena sine lege," the Criminal Law abolished a difference in punishment depending on class, and divided crimes into major, minor, and police offences. On the other hand, the Criminal Procedure Law stipulated the proceedings of a criminal trial or the kind and organization of courts, establishing a system for intermediate and final appeals from district courts to the Supreme Court according to each crime.

Thus, before establishing a constitution, a fundamental law, the national government laid the foundations of the judicial system while countering the people's movement. It was in May 1886 that the government enacted the Regulations for Court Organizations, which addressed the appointment of judges and public prosecutors, their qualifications, tenure for judges, and the relationship of supervision between the judicial branch and the executive branch. After promulgating the Japanese Constitution of 1889 and before the Imperial Diet of 1890 convened, the government enacted the Court Organization Law, the Civil Proceedings Law, and the Code of Criminal Procedure successively. The Attorneys-at-Law Law, which was promulgated in March 1893, is mentioned later.

2. The Age of Institutional Lawyers

(1) The age of institutional daigennin

Lawyers constitute the link between the court and the outside of private law, namely, the community or society. What kind of institutional characteristic did they have?

Lawyers were originally called "*daigennin*"; the first "Regulations as to *Daigennin*" was enacted in 1876. According to the regulations, *daigennin* were familiar with the outlines of decrees, official notices, and their histories; the outlines of criminal law; and the outlines of contemporary legal proceedings. Examined for their conduct or personal history by the local authorities, *daigennin* were certified by the Minister of Justice. This was the beginning of institutional lawyers.

The regulations were revised in May 1880 as follows: A. *Daigennin* shall be supervised by the public prosecutor; B. A legal *daigennin*'s union shall be formed for each of district-court head and branch offices, and *daigennin* shall be recommended to join it — an organization leading to the current bar association. In addition, concerning the examination for *daigennin*, the new regulations stipulated that the Minister of Justice should send the responsible prosecutor the questions — the subjects are law as to civil affairs and criminal matters, legal proceedings, and various regulations for the trial — and the prosecutor should take charge of the examination.

(2) The age of the Attorneys-at-Law Law

The Attorneys-at-Law Law was enforced in May 1893. The Ministry of

Justice had planned to establish law incorporating not only the Court Organization Law but also a three-class system — lawyers belong to the Supreme Court, high courts, or district courts — or expensive license fees and guaranty money. Although this attempt failed, the ministry managed to include the following stipulations in the law: a bar association, one for each district court, shall be closely supervised by the chief public prosecutor; the association cannot discuss matters other than those submitted by the Minister of Justice or courts or those that are related to the judicial branch or the interests of lawyers and about which it memorializes the Ministry of Justice or courts; the association shall be attended by the chief public prosecutor; and the Minister of Justice has authority to declare the association's resolution invalid and stop its proceedings.

Against these official bar associations, the Japan Association of Lawyers was founded in 1896, with the founders including Kazuo Hatoyama; Shiro Isobe, Chair of the Tokyo Bar Association; Tatsuo Kishimoto, who was from Shimane Prefecture, studied abroad in France, and helped found Meiji Law School; and Takeo Kikuchi, who was from Iwate Prefecture, studied abroad in America, and was the first doctor of laws in Japan. This association was intended to facilitate friendship among the members, the progress of the judicial system, and the proper application of law. Once founded, however, it immediately argued for abolishing the preliminary examination or assigning a counsel to the examination. It also discussed the grand jury or the system of public prosecutors.

Later, involving the official bar associations, this connection among lawyers turned out to play a role in subsequent important court battles and influence the quality of court battles in Japan.

(2-1) The Ashio Copper Mine Pollution Case
In the Ashio Copper Mine Pollution Case, the copper mine operated by

Furukawa Mining Industry emitted smoke and toxic gas and discharged water contaminated with minerals, causing enormous damage to residents in the surrounding community. This pollution led to the "Mayhem by Petitioners Wishing to Save Lives," after which fifty-two people were prosecuted for major and minor offenses. For this trial, a defense team of fifty-eight lawyers in total was formed: forty-two from Tokyo and sixteen from Yokohama, Maebashi, and Utsunomiya.

(2-2) The Hibiya Riots
In the Hibiya Riots (mayhem), which erupted on September 5, 1905, in opposition to the peace treaty signed after the Russo-Japanese War, more than 2,000 people were arrested, of whom 313 were prosecuted. While 117 people were found guilty in a preliminary examination and brought to a public trial, 194 were acquitted in the preliminary examination but 2 died. The defendants included three lawyers, who were charged with having masterminded the popular mass meeting.

Taking seriously the fact that the police killed law-abiding citizens, the Tokyo Bar Association divided all Tokyo City into nine areas, assigned each area to its lawyers, fifty-four in total besides the chair, to investigate the incident, and published the results. For the oral proceedings, the association divided the work, assigning general argument to four lawyers, concluding argument to five, and each of the defendants to three–five lawyers. More than 100 lawyers were involved in defending 102 defendants, who were alleged to have been driven by mob psychology. As a result, a large defense team comprising a total of 152 lawyers was formed.

(2-3) The High Treason Incident
The High Treason Incident of 1910 was associated with an assassination plot against the emperor, although it was almost a fabricated incident. The Supreme Court held sixteen trials from December 10 to 29, 1910, behind

closed doors, and handed down its decision with open doors on January 18 next year. For these trials, a total of eleven lawyers tried to defend the accused.

The Japan Association of Lawyers were not only involved in defending the accused in incidents like these. Early in the twentieth century, it also carried on a campaign to transfer the supervision of lawyers and bar associations from the chief public prosecutor to the Minister of Justice. Or it campaigned to place the seat of the lawyer on a level with that of the prosecutor, not parties concerned as was the case. But these campaigns did not succeed. The arrangement of the prosecutor and the judge sitting side by side on a podium was maintained until 1947 after World War II.

(2-4) The Rice Riot
Faced with the Rice Riot of 1918, the Japan Association of Lawyers adopted the following resolution on August 19:
> This riot broke out because food policy by the national government had been insufficient, and the government had not closely investigated the plight of the people. We recognize the need to establish a fundamental policy aiming to swiftly secure the lives of the people. We warn that the government should not take wrong measures in exercising judicial power against the riot.

The association selected sixteen lawyers for a special committee on the food problem, sixteen for a special committee on the riot, sixteen for a special committee on human rights issues, and five for a subcommittee of each special committee. It divided the affected areas into five regions — Shizuoka and Aichi; Yamanashi, Nagano, and Niigata; Hiroshima and Okayama; Kyoto, Osaka, Hyogo, and Mie; and Kyushu — and dispatched lawyers to each region to investigate the incidence, which resulted in a voluminous report. It passed five resolutions criticizing the government for having dispatched the army to the riot or banned carrying articles in newspapers or magazines and giving speeches.

(3) Founding the Japan Lawyers Association for Freedom

Incidents in which lawyers had been involved so far were unorganized mass movements. After the Rice Riot, however, organized and class movements developed, which were oppressed as before. Defense teams of lawyers again played a significant role here. And the defense teams themselves clearly showed their class-oriented nature.

From July to August 1921, the labor union of the Kobe factory of Mitsubishi Shipbuilding and the union of Kawasaki Dockyard staged a strike simultaneously, both demanding eight working hours, the right of collective bargaining for the unions, or the right to join a horizontal union. On July 29, 13,000 laborers of Kawasaki Dockyard gathered at Ikuta Shrine and staged a demonstration. Then, police officers with sword drawn stormed the demonstration, and a laborer was slashed from behind and killed. The Kobe Bar Association entrusted this incidence to a lawyer. On the other hand, the Tokyo Bar Association immediately organized a council to form the Kobe Inquiry Committee into the Violation of Human Rights, and dispatched sixteen committee members to Kobe. They investigated the incidence with the Kobe Bar Association and revealed concrete cases of the violation of human rights, holding meetings to report their findings in Kobe, Osaka, and Tokyo. The "Japan Lawyers Association for Freedom," mainly consisting of these lawyers, was founded around October. The preface of the "Report on the Kobe Human Rights Issues" reads, "Securing rights is the mission of law; the freedom of life and the body is a fundamental right." This phrase was the greatest common denominator among inquiry committee members; the Japan Lawyers Association for Freedom also must have been based on this spirit. Progressives and social democrats rallied in this association.

Encouraged by an atmosphere of Taisho Democracy, proletarian and socialist movements were on the rise, opposing the despotism of the emperor system or its pro-war policy. To oppress these movements, the national government enacted the Peace Preservation Law in 1925. The first wholesale oppression of the Communist Party using this law was the March 15 Incidence in 1928 and the April 16 Incidence next year.

In response, rallying laborers, farmers, and progressive intellectuals, lawyers took the initiative in forming the Victims of Liberation Movements Relief Association. In May 1930, the association became the Japanese branch of the International Laborers' Relief Association (MOPR, commonly known as the "Red Relief Association"), which was founded in 1922.

In addition, to fight court battles associated with the March 15 Incidence or the April 16 Incidence — the first trial was held on June 25, 1931 — the Victims of Liberation Movements Relief Defense Team was formed. While fighting court battles to defend the accused, the team held the funeral of Yoshimichi Iwata or took over the corpse of Takiji Kobayashi, who was killed in prison.

Subsequently, the Defense Team of the National Council for Farmers was formed in 1931; this defense team merged with the Victims of Liberation Movements Relief Defense Team in 1933, forming the Japan Defense Team for Laborers and Farmers. The team's slogans called for A. absolutely opposing class trials led by capitalists and landlords, B. acquitting all offenders against the Peace Preservation Law, C. immediately releasing political prisoners, D. opposing the White Terror, E. opposing the imperialist war, and F. establishing the socialist soviet based on proletarian dictatorship in Japan. The team published the "Social Movement Correspondence," and established branch offices in Tokyo, Yokohama, Mito, Maebashi, Shizuoka, Niigata, Nagoya, Osaka, Fukuoka, Sapporo, Kyongsong, and Tainan.

Afterwards, however, the national government rounded up lawyers belonging to the Japan Defense Team for Laborers and Farmers, and regarded the activity of the team and lawyers itself as committing the "crime of executing the objectives of associations" stipulated in Subsection 1 of Section 1 of the Peace Preservation Law. Moreover, the decision concluding the preliminary examination regarded the Victims of Liberation Movements Relief Defense Team and the Defense Team of the National Council for Farmers as a "secret society" with the aim of expanding and bolstering the Communist Party, and did not allow their continuation. Thus, both the Japan Lawyers Association for Freedom and the Japan Defense Team for Laborers and Farmers were destroyed.

3. Postwar Japanese Society and Justice

(1) The Constitution of Japan and the judicial system after World War II

Japan accepted the Potsdam Declaration and surrendered unconditionally, after it caused tremendous damage to the countries and people of Asia — it killed twenty million people — and its own people in the war over fifteen years. Deeply regretting this war and resolving never to conduct war again, Japan established the Constitution of Japan, which specifies that the right to peacefully live and fundamental human rights are universal human rights, and that sovereignty resides with the people to guarantee these rights. The Japanese people and the Japanese Government declared this constitution to the world, promising to adhere to it. Movements advocating human rights, democracy, and peace in Japan all originate from here.

The Constitution adopts the principle of the separation of powers: legislative power belongs to the Diet (Article 41), executive power to the cabinet (Article 65), and "all judicial power belongs to the Supreme Court and lower courts established in accordance with law" (Article 76, Section

1). In addition, it stipulates that "all judges shall discharge their duties independently according to their conscience and be restricted only by this constitution and law," declaring the independence of judges, that is, the independence of judicial power.

Lower courts below the Supreme Court consist of eight high courts; district courts, one per prefecture; family courts, in the same place as the district court; and 575 summary courts, one per one or two police stations. Among these, the court of first instance is, in principle, the district court, family court, and summary court. The court of second instance is, in principle, the high court. The court of third instance is, again in principle, the Supreme Court. These are all about principles. For example, if a district court tries a civil case of a summary court as the court of second instance, a high court tries the case as the court of third instance. If the defendant makes a special final appeal, the Supreme Court tries the case as the court of fourth instance.

(2) The postwar recovery and pollution problems

Japan started its postwar period in the midst of devastation. As part of the occupation policy by the GHQ, the national government established the Economic Stabilization Agency, which took charge of the economic recovery plan, in August 1946, and decided the "priority production system" in December. Relying on this system, to revive the devastated Japanese economy, the government tried to concentrate funds and materials in key industries such as the coal mining and steel industries, and ultimately boost all production. The Recovery Finance Corporation, which originated from the recovery finance division of the Industrial Bank of Japan, intensively financed the coal mining, steel, electric power, fertilizer, and shipping industries. Among the borrowers was Chisso in Minamata. Chisso, originally named Nippon Nitrogen Fertilizer Corporation, was founded in 1908. It expanded production with the backing of the national war policy, but air raids had destroyed its facilities. After the war, Chisso revived again thanks to support from the national government, which needed to increase the production of fertilizer in parallel with an increase in food production. A company regarding union with the state as the mission of industry takes no account of the possibility of its operation destroying the environment and seriously undermining the health and lives of residents in the surrounding community. In this way, the economic recovery was promoted.

In the period of high economic growth following the recovery period, the environment and health were again largely neglected; pollution problems came to the surface and got serious. Focusing on the expansion of production, companies had hardly invested in measures to improve safety or preserve the environment. Or industrial structure relying largely on the heavy and chemical industries had been established. As a result, air pollution and water pollution by wastewater rapidly got worse mainly in industrial areas. The factory wastewater of Chisso was released into Minamata Bay without any treatment, undermining the lives and health of residents who ate fish and shellfish contaminated with organic mercury on a daily basis.

(3) Polluters, local residents, and justice

To deal with worsening pollution, the national government enacted two laws related to water quality in 1958 and the Smoke Control Law in 1962. However, these laws did not hold back the government's priority on industry; victims or local residents suffering from serious pollution carried on anti-pollution campaigns in various places, which swayed local governments, courts, and the national government.

It was victims in Niigata suffering from so-called second Minamata disease, which was caused by organic mercury — the same causal substance as Minamata disease in Kumamoto — that put pollution on trial for the first time in Japan. The polluter was the Kanose factory of Showa Denko, which released wastewater into the Agano River, causing organic mercury poisoning. The victims filed a lawsuit in the Niigata District Court in September 1967. This battle was followed by a series of lawsuits. In September the same year, victims in Yokkaichi suffering from respiratory disease — the petrochemical complex there caused air

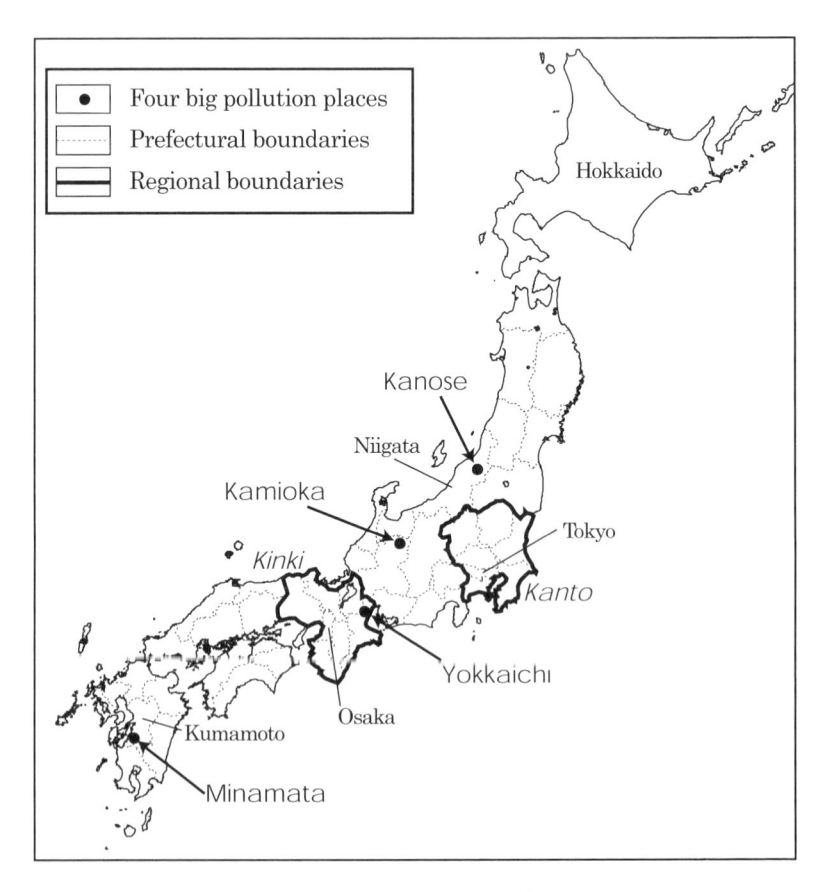

Figure 1. Japan and the four big pollution trials
The area of Kansai roughly corresponds with the Kinki Region.

pollution — filed a lawsuit in the Yokkaichi Branch of the Tsu District Court. In March 1968, victims in Toyama Prefecture suffering from cadmium poisoning — the polluter was the Kamioka mining of Mitsui Kinzoku located upstream along the Jinzu River — filed a lawsuit in the Toyama District Court. And next year, in June 1969, the victims of Minamata disease filed a lawsuit in the Kumamoto District Court.

These are the so-called four big pollution trials. In terms of the extent and scale — it affected an extensive area — the damage of Minamata disease was extremely cruel and severe. But it took a long time for the victims to bring the damage to trial, and they still have to fight. This fact reveals that Minamata disease issues had involved serious problems to be solved with regard to the relationship between the polluter and the community and the relationship between the national government and local governments.

Chisso deeply infiltrated the community and residents of Minamata, forming a relationship neither too close to nor too remote from them in economic and social life. It was also inseparably bound to the Minamata City government. That is why Minamata was called Chisso's castle town. Moreover, this situation was linked to the discriminatory structure of the community. Therefore, it was extremely difficult for victims to voice their criticism of the company.

As a result, the court battle had to be a battle through which victims were freed from various fetters; they had to demonstrate considerable fortitude.

The battle over Minamata disease in the judicial arena was a battle for justice, a battle to achieve the dignity of man and human rights, and a battle fought by victims and various supporters together. In addition, it was waged involving wide-ranging intellectuals and sensible people. And it achieved results step by step. These were major factors in victims themselves fostering independence. It was, however, a group of lawyers that continued to play a pivotal role in connecting these victims with their supporters. The revised "Attorneys-at-Law Law," which was promulgated in 1949, has made it postwar lawyers' duty to "advocate fundamental human rights and realize social justice" (Article 1). Although it is not easy for them to literally stick to this spirit, the group of lawyers has practiced it in the history of battles dating back to the prewar period while involved in Minamata disease issues.

The history of battles centering on Minamata disease issues continues to play an important role in achieving the dignity of man, human rights, and environmental rights — creating an environment where humans and nature can coexist — in postwar Japan.

Chapters 1 to 3 are based on a book originally written in Japanese, ノーモア・ミナマタ 解決版 (Hideo Kitaoka, Kadensha, 2011). The following is the preface to the book.

We concluded the No-More-Minamata Lawsuit Claiming Government Compensation with a victorious settlement in March 2011. We deeply appreciate sympathy and support offered by the public so far.

The 2004 Supreme Court decision on the Kansai Lawsuit recognized those who had eaten large amounts of fish and shellfish from the Shiranui Sea contaminated with mercury released by Chisso and had symptoms like ours as suffering from Minamata disease. Encouraged by this decision, we filed lawsuits demanding relief in the Kumamoto, Tokyo, and Osaka District Courts, and had fought since then over more than five years. It was by no means an easy battle, but thanks to the monolithic solidarity of the plaintiff group and the belief that our demand for relief was justifiable and supported by the public, we managed to overcome one barrier after another.

The goal of the battle stretching over more than five years was to relieve all victims through a judicial relief scheme.

Although we failed to establish a relief scheme applied to victims beyond the plaintiffs, we succeeded in realizing some first attempts in the history of Minamata disease. For example, under the supervision of the court, a third-party committee to which the plaintiffs and the defendants separately nominated the same number of doctors identified eligible patients. Or medical materials submitted by both parties were treated equally. As a result, we paved the way for relieving 94% of 3,000 plaintiffs, or relieving more than 40,000 patients including those relieved by the Law Concerning Special Measures for the Relief of Minamata Disease Victims and the Settlement of Minamata Disease Issues. We are proud of these achievements.

We really feel that there are still many neglected victims in the coastal areas of the Shiranui Sea. Medical examinations of residents in the areas and environmental studies on the whole area of the Shiranui Sea should reveal this fact. Although the trial was concluded, we cannot ignore this fact. We are prepared to strive for relieving all victims.

At the same time as our settlement, the Great East Japan Earthquake occurred, destroying the nuclear power plant and causing unprecedented damage. In unison with the victims of this earthquake, we would like to realize Japan where human life and the environment are respected.

We shall be extremely happy if this booklet forms a small step in that direction.

Toshio Oishi

(Leader of the Plaintiff Group of the No-More-Minamata Lawsuit Claiming Government Compensation)

Chapter 1

The History of Minamata Disease

1. The Outbreak of Minamata Disease

(1) The early history of Minamata disease

Minamata disease is a water pollution disease that broke out in Minamata City, Kumamoto Prefecture, on Japan's southern island of Kyushu. It is called Minamata disease because it broke out in Minamata City. The causal substance is a type of organic mercury, methyl mercury. Methyl mercury was contained in wastewater released from the Minamata factory of Chisso Corporation (Chisso). This methyl mercury was taken by fish and shellfish through the food chain; by eating the fish and shellfish contaminated with methyl mercury, people contracted Minamata disease.

Minamata disease was officially recognized on May 1, 1956. It was also announced in 1965 that the second Minamata disease — Niigata Minamata disease — broke out in Niigata Prefecture in the middle of Japan's central island of Honshu. The polluter in Niigata was the Kanose factory of Showa Denko, which was located upstream along the Agano River.

The conventional measure to prevent pollution is to dilute wastewater discharged from factories. In Minamata, however, it was Minamata Bay that the factory wastewater was released into in the early days. In addition, Minamata Bay is a closed water system in the inland sea, the Shiranui

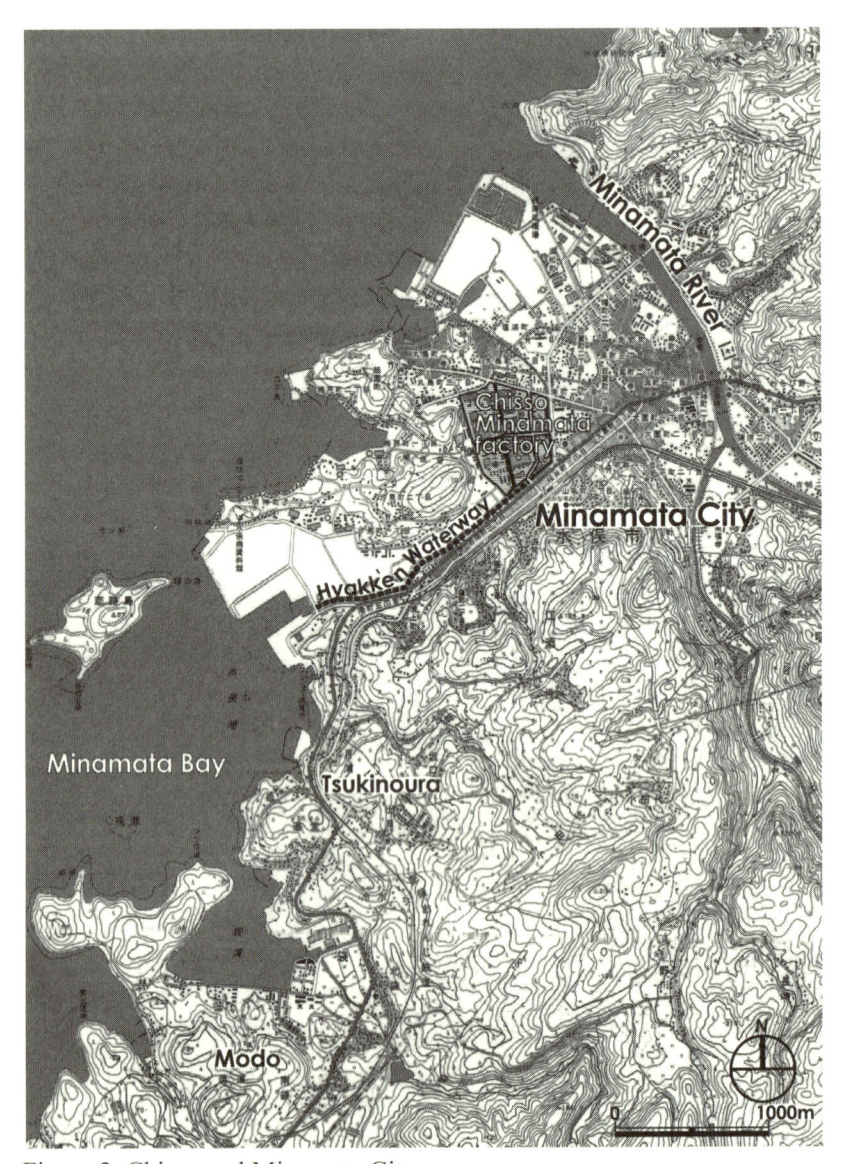

Figure 2. Chisso and Minamata City
This figure is based on the 1:25,000 topographic map (Minamata) published by the Geospatial Information Authority of Japan.

Sea. In Niigata, the Agano River is a closed water system. In both cases, therefore, the factories were located in a closed water system, where methyl mercury was not diluted easily.

In 1908, Chisso built its factory in Minamata, which was a small fishing village on the southern tip of Kumamoto Prefecture. Two years before, Chisso built a power plant nearby in Okuchi, Kagoshima Prefecture. Using abundant electricity generated there and limestone excavated around the Shiranui Sea, it launched the electrochemical industry producing carbide. It subsequently produced ammonia, acetaldehyde, synthetic acetic acid, vinyl chloride, and so on, developing into the leading company in the electrochemical industry in Japan.

As a result of the defeat of Japan in World War II, Chisso had lost all the foreign assets in various places in Asia including the Korean Peninsula and China; the Minamata factory was also severely damaged by American bombing. After the war, however, Chisso rapidly recovered thanks to the support from the national government, transforming Minamata into its "castle town."

Acetaldehyde was produced using mercury, the direct cause for Minamata disease, as a catalyst. Its output amounted to as much as 45,000 tons in 1960, which meant a 25 to 35% share of the national market; Chisso was becoming Japan's leading company.

Around 1950, when Chisso started the mass production of acetaldehyde, various environmental changes started to emerge in the area around Minamata Bay. Something dirty surfaced near the mouth of the wastewater canal in Minamata Bay, and shellfish disappeared. After a while, pollution spread all over the bay. Near the shore of the bay, plenty of fish surfaced or swam staggering; shellfish died with shells open. On land, cats danced madly and killed themselves jumping into the sea; seabirds or crows could not fly any longer and died crawling on the ground. While residents were feeling an ominous presentiment that something wrong was happening in seawater, they nevertheless kept

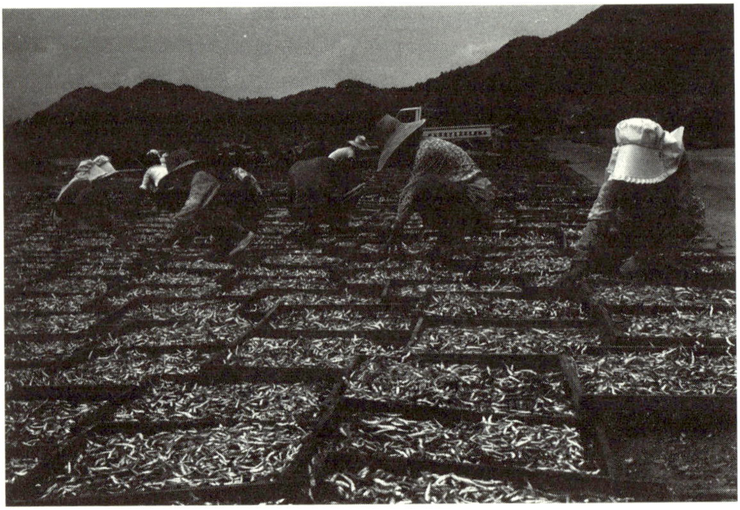

Photo 1. Minamata Bay before Chisso came
Minamata Bay was a "fertile sea." Photo: Hideo Kitaoka

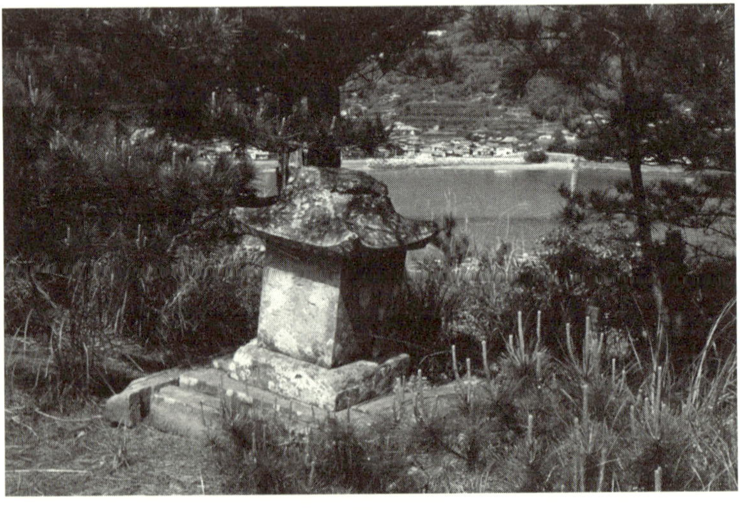

Photo 2. Minamata Bay before Chisso came
Minamata Bay was a "headland where the gods dwelt." Photo: Hideo Kitaoka

catching fish in the sea, eating, and selling it for their livelihoods. On April 21, 1956, a five-year-old daughter of a boatbuilder who also caught fish off the coast of Minamata was admitted to the Chisso factory hospital, which was said to provide the most advanced medical care in the Minamata area in those days. She could not use chopsticks, walked staggering, and could not speak clearly. And it was informed that there were children with similar symptoms in her neighborhood. Confirming this, Hajime Hosokawa, director of the Chisso factory hospital, reported to the Minamata Public Health Center on May 1, "cryptogenic patients with a chief complaint of brain symptoms appeared; four of them were hospitalized." Later, this day was regarded as the day when Minamata disease was officially recognized.

In response to this report, organizations concerned, including the local medical association, formed a task force, which reviewed clinical charts kept in local medical facilities. It turned out that again a five-year-old girl had contracted the disease in December 1953. This patient is regarded as the first patient of Minamata disease. But the production of acetaldehyde using mercury as a catalyst started in 1932. Therefore some point out that the disease had in fact started earlier, although people had overlooked it without knowing what it was.

(2) Studying the cause of the disease

To respond to the outbreak of the serious "strange disease," Kumamoto University organized a study group, whose members were mainly from the School of Medicine. The study group hospitalized the patients as subjects for study and conducted an epidemiological study and autopsies. As a result, it found out that "the causal substance is some sort of heavy metal," which entered the human body through "fish and shellfish." If appropriate measures had been taken at this stage — banning the consumption of fish and shellfish, for example — on the grounds that

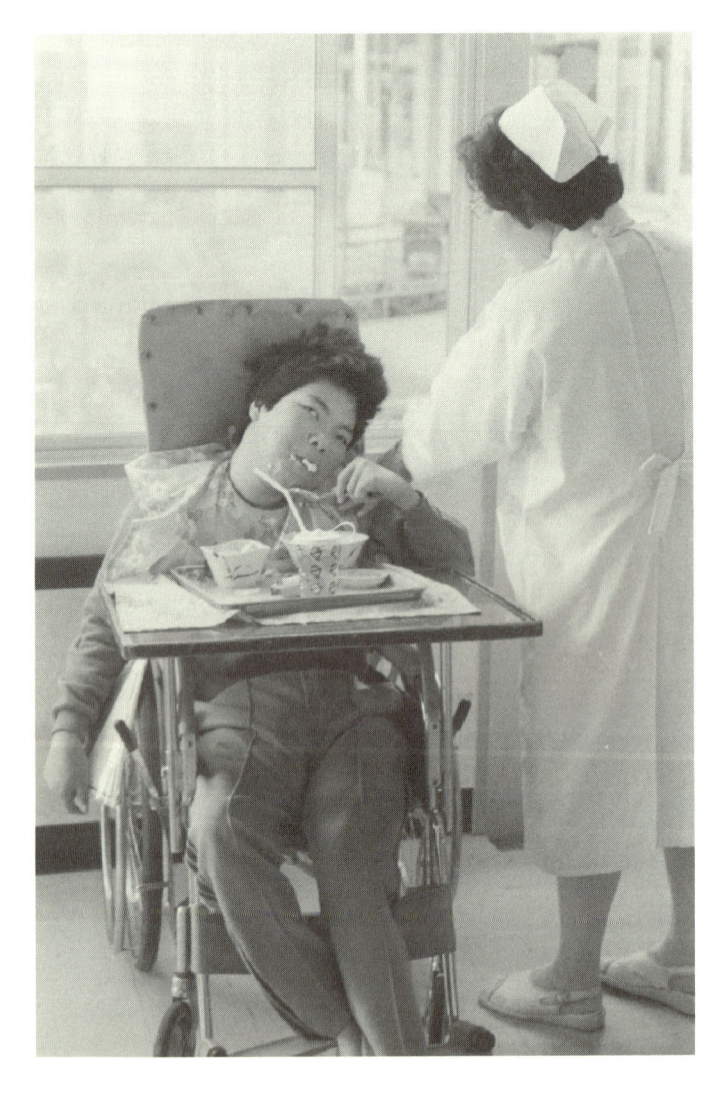

Photo 3. Meisuien, a special hospital for Minamata disease
Photo: Hideo Kitaoka

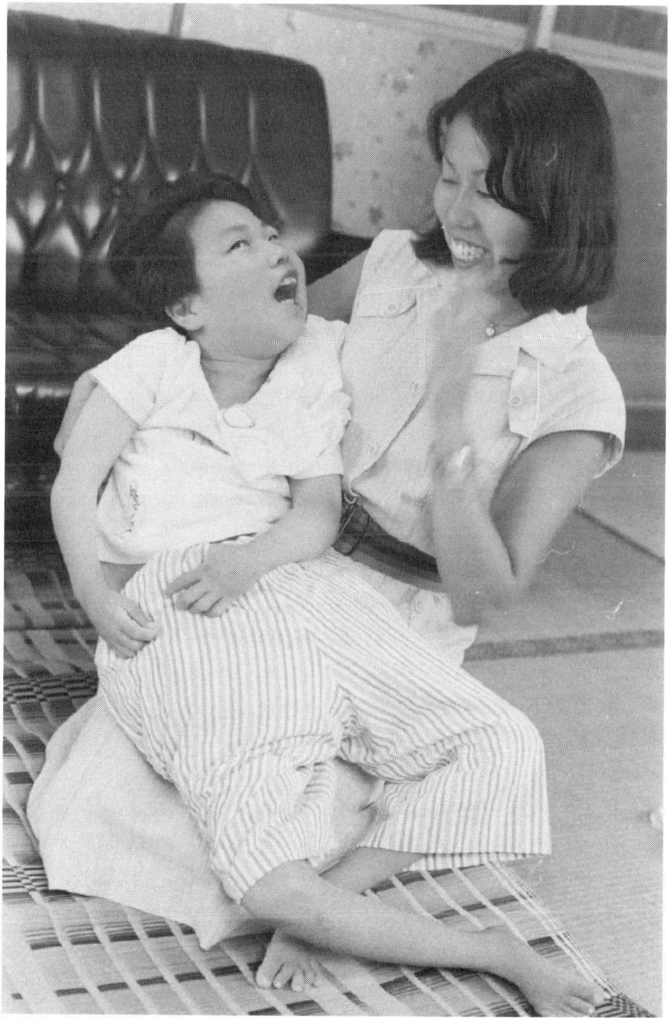

Photo 4. Minamata disease victim
Itsuko Fukuda died at the age of twelve without being certified as a Congenial Minamata disease victim. Photo. Hideo Kitaoka

substances harmful to the human body were causing the disease through fish and shellfish, then the increase of patients would have been prevented, even if the causal substance had not been identified or the mechanism of the onset of the disease had not been understood. This was the first and biggest blunder committed by the national and prefectural governments.

The Chisso Minamata factory was suspected to be the source of the contamination, but it continued to release untreated wastewater containing organic mercury.

Finally in July 1959, the study group of Kumamoto University announced that organic mercury was the causal substance. Chisso immediately refuted, saying that the organic mercury theory presented by the study group was "wrong in terms of scientific common sense." In addition, various organizations or individuals refuted or obstructed the group's work: the Japan Chemical Industry Association, of which Chisso was a member, announced, "the disease was caused by having dumped explosives after World War II"; or a researcher enlisted by the national government put forward the "Amino poisoning theory."

In November 1959, the Minamata Food Poisoning Special Committee of the Ministry of Health and Welfare's Food Sanitation Investigation Council, which mainly consisted of members of the study group of Kumamoto University, submitted to the Minister of Health and Welfare a report stating, "the major causative agent of Minamata disease is some sort of organic mercury compound contained in fish and shellfish in Minamata Bay." The next day, however, the ministry dissolved this committee because it did not want to accept this report. While refuting the study group of Kumamoto University, Chisso itself in fact was conducting the "cat experiment" secretly, in which cats were fed food mixed with the factory wastewater. And a cat, called no. 400, manifested the symptoms of Minamata disease in October 1959. But Chisso kept this fact absolutely secret, insisting that the cause of the disease was unknown.

The History of Minamata Disease

In this way, Chisso, the Japan Chemical Industry Association, and the Ministry of Health and Welfare covered up the fact, and refuted and obstructed the work of the study group of Kumamoto University to find out the cause of the disease.

The study group, however, continued its work. It extracted the crystal of an organic mercury compound from shellfish from Minamata Bay next year. Furthermore, it isolated methyl mercury chloride from the mercury dregs of Chisso's acetaldehyde plant in August 1962, plunging an inescapable scientific scalpel. A scientific conclusion was reached in February 1963: the group announced, "Minamata disease is a toxic disease caused by eating fish and shellfish from Minamata Bay. The causal substance is a methyl mercury compound," which "was isolated from shellfish from Minamata Bay as well as from the sludge of the Chisso Minamata factory." This was the result of strenuous efforts by university researchers who searched for truth.

On the other hand, concerning the response of the national government, it — the Ministry of Health and Welfare — set about investigating the cause of the disease at the beginning of its outbreak. But once Chisso came under investigation, the government rather tried to cover up the cause.

When the heavy metal poisoning theory was announced in 1956, the Kumamoto prefectural government inquired of the ministry whether it "[could] ban the capture of fish and shellfish by applying the Food Sanitation Law." Because the national and prefectural governments had to compensate losses fifty-fifty, the ministry replied, "because there is no clear evidence that all fish and shellfish from Minamata Bay are contaminated, the Food Sanitation Law cannot be applied." Nor did the ministry apply the Water Quality Control Law and the Factory Effluent Control Law, both of which were enacted in 1958, leaving Chisso to release untreated wastewater. It was not until September 1968, after acetaldehyde factories had disappeared in Japan, that the ministry and the

Science and Technology Agency, that is, the national government admitted that Minamata disease was "a pollution-related disease caused by the Chisso Minamata factory."

(3) Chisso's insincere response to victims

Because Chisso released the factory wastewater without treating it, Chisso polluted the sea from the beginning of its operation. The pollution became serious gradually, and a compensation agreement was signed between Chisso and the Minamata Fishing Cooperative as early as 1926. But it was in 1956, when the disease was officially recognized, that the outbreak of the disease came to the surface.

Subsequently, Chisso continued to increase the production of acetaldehyde; patients increased proportionately with it. The Minamata Fishing Cooperative demanded compensation or investigation into the cause. So Chisso changed the wastewater output route: wastewater was now released not into the Hyakken Waterway, which poured wastewater into seriously polluted Minamata Bay, but into the Minamata River via the Yahata Pool at the mouth of the river. Surprised at this change, the national government forced Chisso to bring the output route back to the Hyakken Waterway in November 1959. Therefore, because Chisso kept increasing the production of acetaldehyde without taking any measure against the source of the contamination, the outbreak of Minamata disease spread across the Shiranui Sea.

On December 30, 1959, Chisso signed the first agreement with a victims' group through the mediation of the Kumamoto prefectural governor. But this was not a compensation agreement; this was called a "sympathy money agreement," which assumed that the cause was unknown and stipulated that Chisso should express sympathy with victims. In fact, Chisso had already known that it was the culprit for the outbreak of the disease thanks to the above-mentioned "cat experiment."

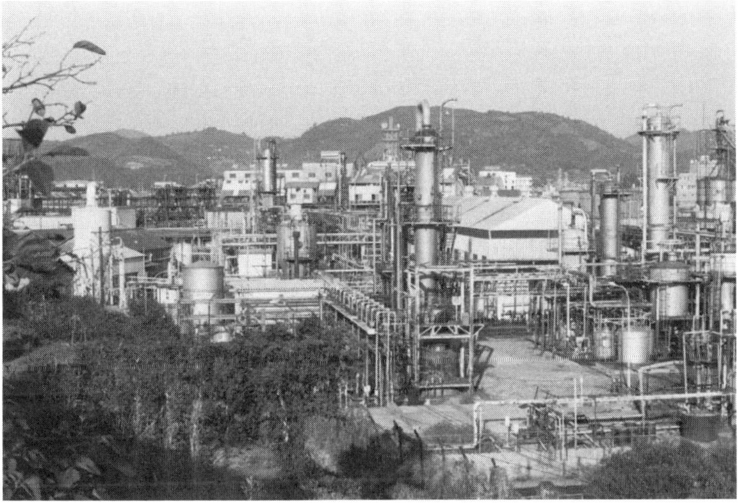

Photo 5. Polluter Chisso Minamata factory
Photo: Hideo Kitaoka

The content of the agreement was extremely unfair: 1) the money was insufficient, 300,000 yen for a dead patient, for example; 2) Chisso will not pay further compensation even if it is identified as the culprit for Minamata disease; and 3) Chisso will stop paying this money if it turns out that Chisso is not the culprit.

But patients, who could not work because of the disease and struggled to pay for livelihoods as well as medical care, finally signed this agreement. Later, the decision on the First Kumamoto Minamata Disease Lawsuit found that this agreement offended against public order and decency and was invalid, stating, "the agreement stipulated an extremely small amount of money taking advantage of patients' ignorance and poverty, and forced patients to give up their claims for damages."

Given the organic mercury theory presented by the study group of Kumamoto University in July 1959, the fishermen of Minamata pressed Chisso to treat its factory wastewater. In response, Chisso installed the

Cyclator, a water purification system, in December the same year, announcing that its wastewater was purified thanks to this system and that the outbreak of Minamata disease would end. At the press conference at the ceremony for the completion of the Cyclator, the factory manager demonstratively drank a glass of water that was allegedly wastewater treated through the system. But later, it turned out that the water had been just tap water while the Cyclator had been neither intended for nor capable of removing mercury. After all, Chisso kept releasing organic mercury, the causal substance of Minamata disease, without treating wastewater until 1966, when the complete circular system was introduced. Chisso stopped the production of acetaldehyde in May 1968; four months later, the national government admitted for the first time that Minamata disease was a pollution-related disease caused by Chisso.

2. The Progress of Trials

(1) From the First Kumamoto Minamata Disease Lawsuit to the Third Lawsuit

In the Minamata area, which was called Chisso's castle town, it was not easy to hold Chisso responsible for the disease, even if people knew that the disease was caused by wastewater from the Chisso factory. Faced with Chisso continuously responding insincerely, however, patients decided to go to court, which was, in their view, the only way to restore damage fairly.

The main point of contention in the First Kumamoto Minamata Disease Lawsuit, which was filed in June 1969, was whether the court would recognize Chisso's liability for negligence. The Kumamoto District Court handed down its decision on March 20, 1973, which condemned Chisso, recognized its liability, found the above-mentioned sympathy

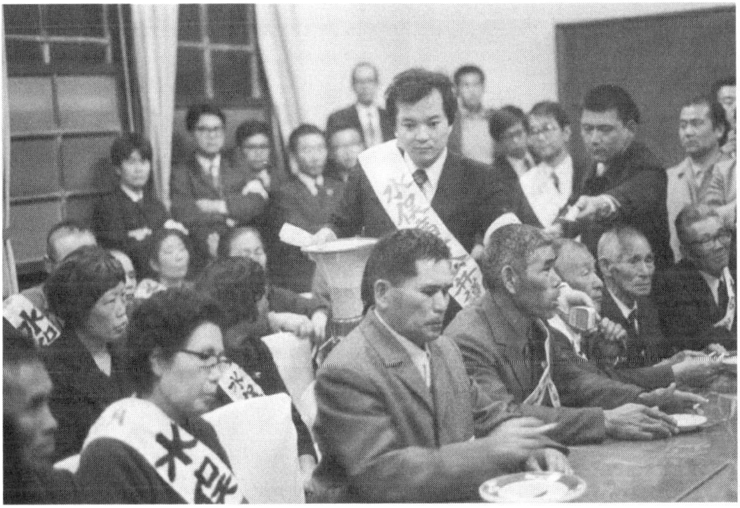

Photo 6. First Kumamoto Minamata Disease Lawsuit
In the First Kumamoto Minamata Disease Lawsuit, plaintiffs fought claiming the right to live in peace, keeping in mind their grief and suffering and the regret of those who had passed away. Photo: Hideo Kitaoka

money agreement offensive to public order and decency and invalid, and ordered Chisso to pay 16 million to 18 million yen in compensation for each patient. After this epoch-making decision, Chisso signed compensation agreements with victims' groups, and provisional disposition for governments to remove sludge in Minamata Bay was approved. Moreover, the president of Chisso was found guilty in the criminal trial.

The Second Kumamoto Minamata Disease Lawsuit was filed in January 1973, and led to the relief of as-yet-uncertified patients. In those days, the national government adopted a "policy of abandoning large numbers of victims": it used strict criteria to certify patients as suffering from Minamata disease; or the certification committee consisted of medical doctors selected by the government. These criteria were called the "1977 Certification Criteria," which required a combination of multiple symptoms for the certification of the disease while refusing to certify patients only with sensory disorders. Concerning the Second Lawsuit, the Kumamoto District Court handed down its decision in March 1979, which did not adopt these criteria and certified twelve of fourteen victims as Minamata disease sufferers.

In addition, the decision by the Fukuoka High Court in August 1985 certified victims as suffering from Minamata disease, if they met epidemiological conditions, such as eating large amounts of contaminated fish, even if they exhibited only sensory disorders in all four extremities. This decision criticized the national government's strict criteria and the certification committee, stating, "the government's criteria for certification are failing." These lawsuits highlighted problems with the government's "policy of abandoning large numbers of victims."

Despite these successive decisions in favor of victims, the national government — the Environment Agency — did not revise the criteria for certification. Plaintiffs and the defense team considered that, for the relief of patients, it was necessary to change the national policy by establishing the responsibility of the national government. They launched the Third Kumamoto Minamata Disease Lawsuit in May 1980 to hold the national and Kumamoto prefectural governments responsible. This lawsuit involved large numbers of plaintiffs — 1,400 people — suing in the Kumamoto District Court. It also carried on a nationwide campaign: the lawsuit was filed in Niigata, Tokyo, Kyoto, and Fukuoka as well, and the national liaison council was formed. The Kumamoto District Court handed down its decision on the First Part of the Third Lawsuit in March 1987; the court found the national and Kumamoto prefectural governments responsible, giving a complete victory to plaintiffs. Afterwards, the Tokyo District Court issued a recommendation for settlement in September 1990; other district courts followed suit. The draft scheme of the settlement proposed by the Fukuoka High Court included allowances for medical treatment and care provided through the

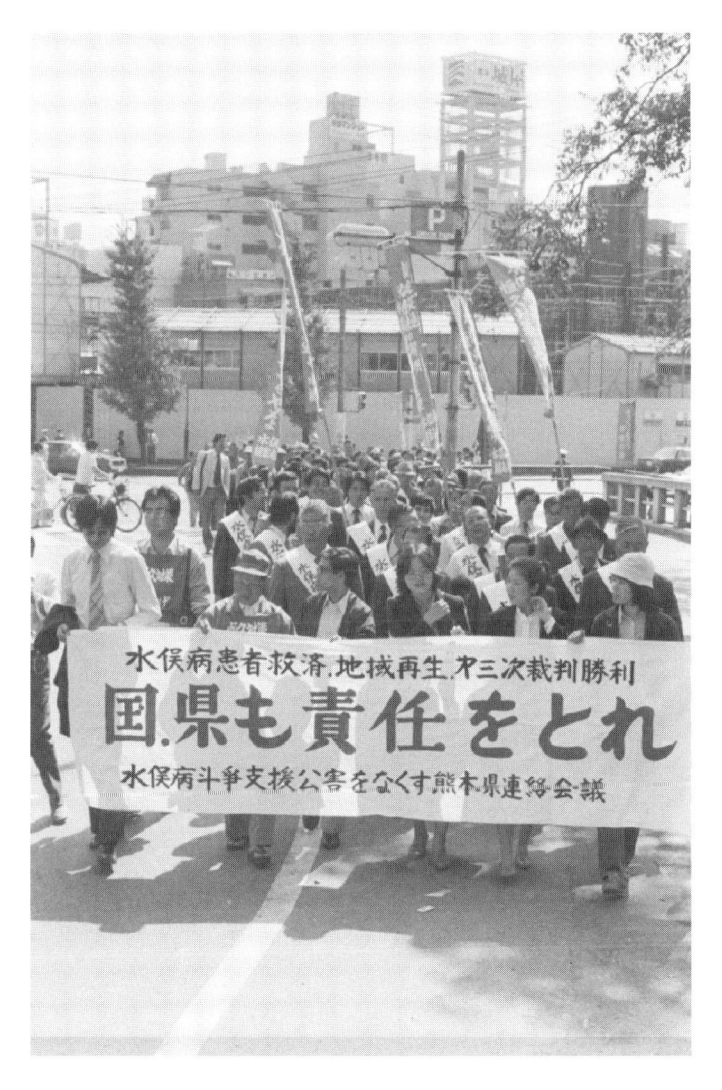

Photo 7. Third Kumamoto Minamata Disease Lawsuit
"The polluter Chisso is of course to blame; the national and prefectural governments, which tried to cover up the crime, are equally to blame! Take responsibility!" Overcoming grief and regret, plaintiffs were determined not to allow the same fault to be committed again. Photo: Hideo Kitaoka

comprehensive medical care project and a lump-sum payment — 8 million yen, 6 million yen, and 4 million yen, respectively. But the national government rejected this scheme.

The national and Kumamoto prefectural governments were again found responsible by the Kumamoto District Court in its decision on the Second Part of the Third Lawsuit in March 1993 and the Kyoto District Court in its decision in November the same year. Both of these courts judged, "if patients meet epidemiological conditions and exhibit sensory disorders in the distal portion of all four extremities, and their symptoms cannot be explained by other diseases, then they should be certified as Minamata disease sufferers." Although district courts or the Fukuoka High Court repeatedly ruled that the strict criteria of the national government did not work, the government has not changed its policy.

Faced with a succession of the district court decisions finding the national government responsible, it was forced to respond, and proposed the draft of the Final Solution Scheme in December 1995. The plaintiff group accepted this next year and also signed an agreement with Chisso. This 1995 political solution did not clearly recognize patients as Minamata disease sufferers, leaving the responsibility of the national and Kumamoto prefectural governments vague. Considering the aging of plaintiffs, and to achieve the swift relief of large numbers of plaintiffs, however, 11,000 patients chose to accept the political solution. These patients included the plaintiffs of the No More Minamata Disease National Liaison Council of Victims and Defense Teams, which was to be formed later.

(2) The Supreme Court decision on the Kansai Lawsuit in October 2004 and subsequent development

On the other hand, the plaintiff group of the Kansai Lawsuit, which was formed by Minamata disease patients who had once lived around

Minamata Bay and moved to Kansai, pursued not the political solution but the ruling in court consistently.

In its decision on the Kansai Lawsuit on April 27, 2001, the Osaka High Court found not only Chisso but also the national and Kumamoto prefectural governments responsible, and certified patients as Minamata disease sufferers if they presented sensory disorders. On October 15, 2004, the Supreme Court supported the decision by the Osaka High Court, establishing the responsibility of the national and Kumamoto prefectural governments. Concerning the clinical picture of Minamata disease, the Supreme Court endorsed the 2001 judgment by the Osaka High Court.

The judgment by the Osaka High Court certifies methyl mercury poisoning by using the following criteria:

    1) there is proof that a patient ate large amounts of contaminated fish and shellfish from around Minamata Bay;

    2) a patient who meets either of the following three requirements:

        a) a patient who has disorders in two-point discrimination on the tip of the tongue or a patient who has disorders in two-point discrimination on the tip of the finger and shows no influence from constriction of neck vertebrae;

        b) a patient who has certified patients within the family and has sensory disorders in the distal portion of all four extremities;

        c) if a patient was not examined for two-point discrimination for some reason such as death, a patient who had sensory disorders around the mouth or concentric constriction of the visual field.

That is why the Supreme Court approved the Osaka High Court having based its judgment about Minamata disease only on sensory disorders.

It had been assumed that problems with Minamata disease were settled by the 1995 political solution. But the 2004 Supreme Court decision on the Kansai Lawsuit brought about an utterly different situation. For the decision certified patients as Minamata disease sufferers by applying less strict criteria than those of the national government. As a result, applicants for the certification increased rapidly, expecting that the criteria of the government would be revised, so that they could receive relief.

But the national government — the Ministry of the Environment — did not try to revise its criteria, making the excuse that "the Supreme Court decision [did] not directly deny the criteria." After all, despite a series of lawsuits and even the Supreme Court decision, the government revealed a stance firmly rejecting the fundamental relief of Minamata disease patients. Faced with such a stance of the government, Minamata disease patients once again recognized that the government would not change its policy outside court; among them, those who tried to realize relief by directly suing the government increased.

On October 3, 2005, a plaintiff group formed by fifty members of a victims' group, the Association of Minamata Disease Victims "SHIRANUI" (Association "SHIRANUI"), filed the "No-More-Minamata Lawsuit Claiming Government Compensation" against the national and Kumamoto prefectural governments and Chisso in the Kumamoto District Court.

Chapter 2
The Record of Battle in the No-More-Minamata Lawsuit Claiming Government Compensation

1. The Aim of the Lawsuit

The No-More-Minamata Lawsuit Claiming Government Compensation aimed to realize the swift relief of large numbers of victims by using the judicial system. The above-mentioned "1995 political solution" relieved about 10,000 victims. Nevertheless, there still remained many neglected victims, it was estimated. For a comprehensive study on pollution had not been conducted, although about 200,000 people lived in the coastal areas of the Shiranui Sea when the sea was heavily polluted; many of them must have eaten large amounts of contaminated fish and shellfish from around Minamata Bay. In addition, victims were subjected to slanders such as a "bogus patient asking for money"; they were still reluctant to come forward for fear of discrimination and prejudice.

But, because the 2004 Supreme Court decision on the Kansai Lawsuit was handed down and it revised the criteria for certification, expectations grew that victims could receive relief, which led many victims to apply for certification. Despite this Supreme Court decision, however, the national government did not revise the criteria, nor did it take sufficient measures for relief. Although the swift relief of tens of thousands of victims should be in principle addressed through legislative or executive

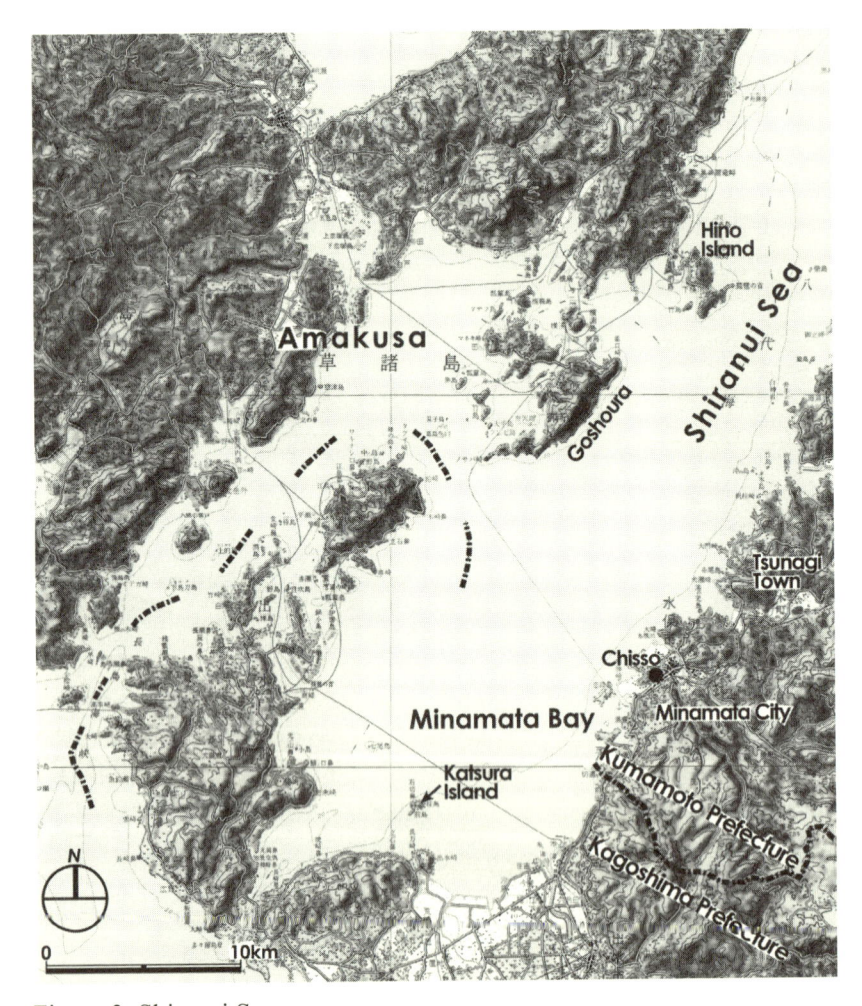

Figure 3. Shiranui Sea
This figure is based on the 1:200,000 regional map (Yatsushiro) published by the Geospatial Information Authority of Japan.

measures, such measures were not taken.

Backed by the Association "SHIRANUI," the first fifty plaintiffs filed a lawsuit claiming compensation in the Kumamoto District Court on October 3, 2005. From the beginning, the plaintiffs aimed to achieve the swift relief of large numbers of victims through a judicial settlement. For most victims were old and there were possibly tens of thousands of neglected victims; solving through rulings was expected to take several decades, with the unreasonable result that victims were not relieved while in life.

An out-of-court settlement tends to be regarded as a solution that adds the two together and divides by two. This is by no means the case with Minamata disease. In the history of lawsuits over Minamata disease, the national government had never entered into settlement negotiations. In the Third Minamata Disease Lawsuit, for example, the plaintiffs carried on a desperate campaign, staging a sit-in for several days in front of the

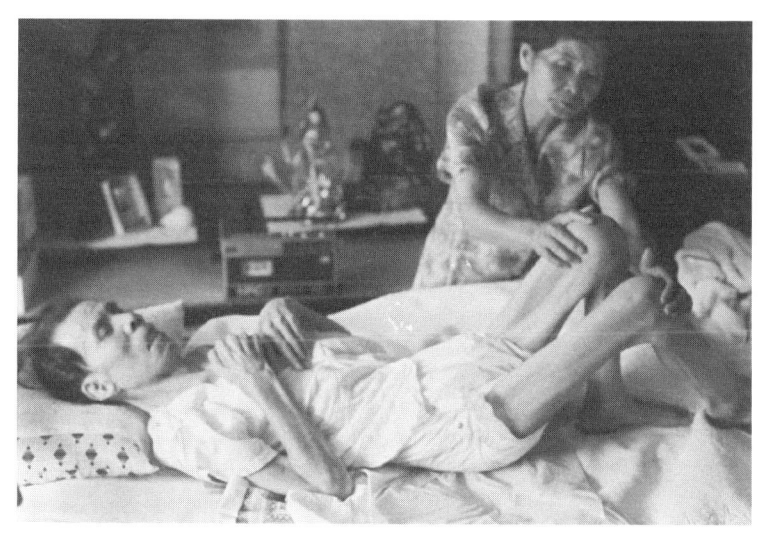

Photo 8. Minamata disease victim
Refusing to be hospitalized, Yahei Ikeda died at home in the season when white flowers bloomed in the garden. Photo: Hideo Kitaoka

prime minister's official residence, under the slogan, "relief while in life." But the national government persistently refused to enter into settlement negotiations. It had been extremely difficult just to force the government to the negotiating table.

The national government had rejected an out-of-court settlement because of the theory of the foundation of governance — the view that, because the responsibility for government compensation and the criteria for certification are related to the foundation of governance, these issues cannot be addressed in settlement negotiations. We, the plaintiffs, thought that this theory had lost its basis in the wake of the 2004 Supreme Court decision; we reached the conclusion that the only way to achieve the swift relief of tens of thousands of victims was a judicial settlement. Our strategy was to thoroughly prove the accuracy of medical certificates issued by a team of medical doctors in court; press the national government to resolve Minamata disease issues by filing mass lawsuits; lead a court to issue a recommendation for settlement; and reach a basic agreement after negotiations, realizing a settlement.

When the First Part of the No-More-Minamata Lawsuit was filed, the then Minister of the Environment immediately rejected an out-of-court settlement. The plaintiffs felt very sad, but fought the battle over five and a half years, backed by broad support and encouragement. Finally they realized a basic agreement in March 2010, and a settlement in March 2011.

2. The Record of the Court Battle

(1) Campaigns for increasing plaintiffs and maintaining solidarity

Our trial started when the above-mentioned first fifty, that is, the plaintiff group of the First Part filed a lawsuit in the Kumamoto District Court on

October 3, 2005. Subsequently, the plaintiff group of the Second Part, 503 plaintiffs, filed a lawsuit on November 14 the same year; our trial turned into a mammoth lawsuit.

In the case of Minamata disease, however, there were some victims' groups locally, of which the Association "SHIRANUI" — which backed the plaintiff group of the No-More-Minamata Lawsuit — was not the largest in membership. In addition, among these victims' groups, those that tried to seek fair compensation in court were not in the majority.

When our trial started, the then Minister of the Environment said, "we won't seek a settlement with the plaintiffs," indicating confidence in the trial. For, among victims' groups that sought relief outside court, there were some groups that were prepared to accept relief measures presented by the national government, and victims who belonged to these groups had an advantage in number.

Our battle started with relaxing such a firm stance of the government and transforming our plaintiff group into a "negotiation partner far from being negligible" to the government.

(1-1) Campaigns under the slogan, the "relief of all Minamata disease victims"

Toshio Oishi, chair of the Association "SHIRANUI" and leader of the plaintiff group of the No-More-Minamata Lawsuit, always advocated the "relief of all Minamata disease victims." Under this slogan, we insisted that our battle was exactly one leading to the relief of all victims, and increased the members of the Association "SHIRANUI" and plaintiffs in the No-More-Minamata Lawsuit.

There was always not enough information for Minamata disease victims. Particularly concerning current Minamata disease, there were some compensation schemes while stances of victims' groups were diverse. Under this situation, seeking accurate information, those who suspected that they also had the symptoms of Minamata disease joined the Association "SHIRANUI" in large numbers.

But not all those who joined the Association "SHIRANUI" became plaintiffs in the No-More-Minamata Lawsuit.

"Going to court" required extraordinary courage from victims. We started a house-to-house visit with the members of the Association "SHIRANUI" from January 2009 so that, overcoming such reluctance, many of them became plaintiffs. We called this campaign "Joint 2009," aiming to increase the number of plaintiffs from about 1,500 at the beginning of the campaign to 2,000 in around half a year. At the same time, we realized a lawsuit in the Osaka District Court, which was mainly brought by victims who lived in the Kinki Region. To increase plaintiffs, we conducted the house-to-house visit with the members of the Association "SHIRANUI," organized local meetings, and asked the plaintiffs to invite their relatives, friends, and acquaintances with the symptoms of Minamata disease into the trial. In addition, we delivered all homes a leaflet urging locals to undergo a medical examination or conducted an advertising campaign on the streets, striving to uncover hidden victims who had not yet been able to come forward.

We presumed that there also remained many neglected victims in the Amakusa area "across the sea," which we had not addressed so far. So we arranged an explanatory meeting about the trial for residents on Hino Island of Ryugatake Town in Kamiamakusa City on April 1 the same year. More than one hundred, presumably most of the residents, participated in the meeting, listening closely to the explanation of the trial. Subsequently, we held meetings repeatedly at various places. The meeting on Hino Island made us painfully aware of the necessity to uncover victims in the Amakusa area. As a result of these campaigns, we were able to increase the number of plaintiffs to about 1,900 by the end of July 2009.

It was medical examinations of residents in the coastal areas of the Shiranui Sea — the Mass Medical Examinations — in September 2009 that led to a dramatic increase in the number of plaintiffs. The Mass

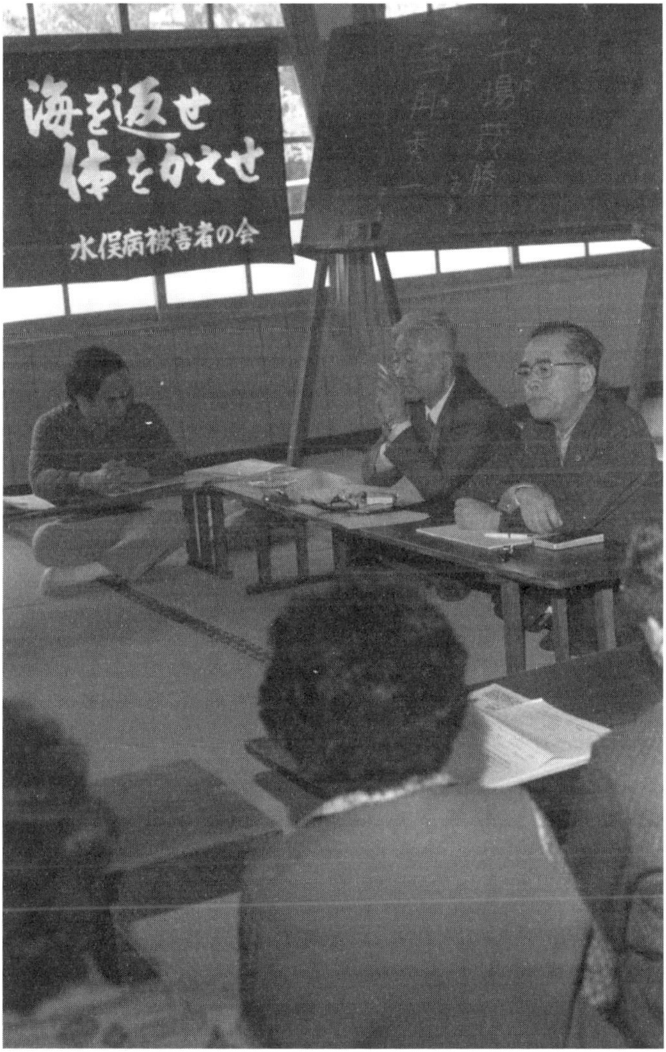

Photo 9. Meeting of victims
Minamata disease victims' groups have demanded to "Return the sea! Return the body!" in order to prevent Minamata from being repeated. Photo: Hideo Kitaoka

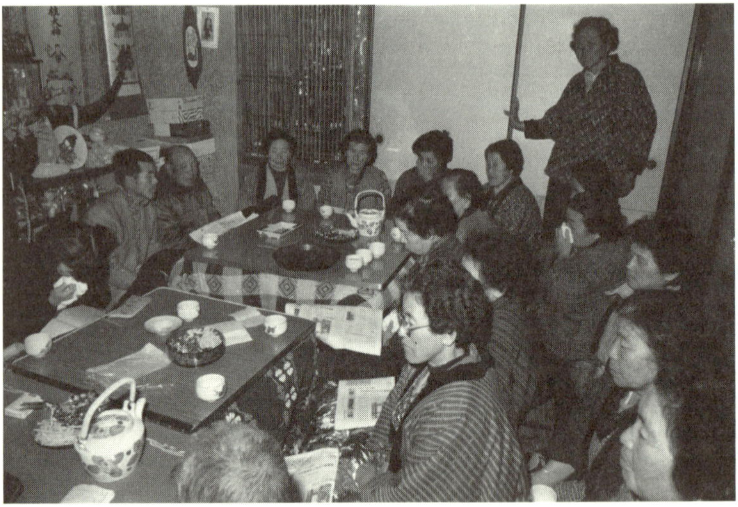

Photo 10. Meeting of victims
Minamata disease victims' groups hold meetings again and again — which are held for each neighborhood in dozens of places — hoping not to repeat Minamata. Photo: Hideo Kitaoka

Medical Examinations was carried out by a committee consisting of seven Minamata disease victims' groups; the team of medical doctors of the Minamata Disease Citizens' Council; the Japan Federation of Democratic Medical Institutions; volunteers from local medical associations, and so on. The chair of the committee was Masazumi Harada, professor at Kumamoto Gakuen University. Among others, the Association "SHIRANUI" made a broad appeal for people to undergo the examinations and collected examinees also in the Amakusa area.

At the Mass Medical Examinations, about 140 doctors gathered from all over the country; as many as about 600 health care workers participated in the event. These doctors and health care workers were allocated to seventeen venues in Kumamoto and Kagoshima Prefectures, where about 1,000 people in total underwent examinations on September 20 and 21, 2009. The Mass Medical Examinations yielded abundant fruit:

many hidden victims recognized their symptoms, which led them to seek compensation. But the fruit of the examinations was not limited to this. Because many doctors and health care workers gathered at the Mass Medical Examinations from across the country, the diagnosis of Minamata disease was better understood throughout the country, which resulted in a lawsuit in Tokyo. Or the examinations led to an increase in medical facilities where victims who had moved to distant places from the coastal areas of the Shiranui Sea, such as Tokyo or Osaka, could undergo medical examinations of the disease or receive treatment; these facilities provided great support for victims.

After the Mass Medical Examinations, we organized many explanatory meetings about the trial at various places, stressing that the trial was the only way to secure fair compensation. These meetings were especially convincing to victims in areas where they could not receive the health notebooks or the treatment notebooks for the Minamata Disease Certification Applicants' Research and Treatment Project because of geographical demarcation by governments. The latter notebooks are issued to applicants for Minamata disease certification, in principle, a year after they apply so that their medical expenses are compensated until the certification committee reaches a conclusion. These victims decided to file a lawsuit, trusting their last hopes to the trial. As a result, we succeeded in passing the 2,000-plaintiff mark on November 18, 2009, after the Mass Medical Examinations.

In this way, while we increased the number of plaintiffs, we repeatedly organized meetings locally and maintained solidarity among plaintiffs, fostering belief in the trial in the mind of each plaintiff.

(1-2) The battle against the attempt to split the plaintiff group
From the end of 2008 to 2009, the Government Parties' Project Team for Minamata Disease Issues came up with measures extremely insufficient in terms of the level of relief. In addition, the Diet passed the Law

Concerning Special Measures for the Relief of Minamata Disease Victims and the Settlement of Minamata Disease Issues on July 8, 2009, which was mainly intended to divide Chisso. Thus the national government tried to split the plaintiff group.

But the plaintiff group was not split by this. We defeated the government's intention by increasing the number of plaintiffs and strengthening the solidarity of the plaintiff group. The government was threatened by the fact that we kept increasing the number of plaintiffs regardless of geographical demarcation by governments while we maintained the solidarity of the plaintiff group without yielding to any attempt to split the group. The plaintiff group had become "a group the government could not ignore" any more.

The government must have been threatened particularly by the fact that many victims joined in the trial in the Amakusa area, where it had been assumed there were no victims of Minamata disease. For the government could not predict how widely victims appeared. To stop the momentum of the plaintiff group, the government could not but negotiate with the plaintiff group and conclude the trial quickly.

By striving for the "increase" and "solidarity" in this way, we succeeded in changing the stance of the government, which had declared, "we won't seek a settlement with the plaintiffs." As a consequence, the trial entered into settlement negotiations, and the level of relief based on the Law Concerning Special Measures was also substantially agreed upon in the trial.

Subsequently, a lawsuit was also filed in the Tokyo District Court, spreading the battle nationwide. The plaintiff group had in fact become a group leading Minamata disease victims.

(2) The points of contention and the lawsuit

(2-1) The clinical picture as the point of contention
In the No-More-Minamata Lawsuit, the main point of contention was "whether each of the plaintiffs [was] a Minamata disease sufferer." To be specific, this point of contention can be divided into the following three questions:

    a) What kind of disease is Minamata disease in reality? (the symptoms of Minamata disease)

    b) Given this reality, how are victims diagnosed as suffering from Minamata disease? (the method for examination or the criteria for diagnosis)

    c) In light of the criteria for diagnosis, can each of the plaintiffs be diagnosed as suffering from Minamata disease?

The questions a) and b) — the general theory of the clinical picture — are relevant to all the plaintiffs; the question c) — the specific theory of the clinical picture — is relevant to the individual plaintiff.

(2-2) Making a uniform medical certificate
The number of plaintiffs in the No-More-Minamata Lawsuit exceeded 1,000 in April 2006, and was expected to increase subsequently.

We were afraid that it would take overwhelmingly long for the court to judge whether each of so many plaintiffs suffered from Minamata disease. Therefore, we argued that a "uniform medical certificate," which used a uniform method for examination and a uniform format, would make a rapid and appropriate judgment possible. Advocated by Prof. Masazumi Harada, who taught Minamata issues at Kumamoto Gakuen University, the uniform medical certificate was a medical certificate for Minamata disease. It was created through thorough consideration by those interested, such as medical doctors, who had been involved in the treatment and research of Minamata disease patients for a long time.

These individuals had only one wish: they wanted to realize the swift and appropriate relief of Minamata disease victims by creating the uniform medical certificate for Minamata disease. Their effort resulted in a) the criteria for the diagnosis of Minamata disease, b) the uniform procedure for examination necessary for the diagnosis, and c) the format of the medical certificate.

That is why the uniform medical certificate should be regarded as a culmination concerning the diagnosis of current Minamata disease.

This certificate has three characteristics as follows.

First, this presents not criteria for the diagnosis of methyl mercury poisoning in general, but criteria for the diagnosis of Minamata disease as a pollution-related disease caused by enormous environmental pollution resulting from wastewater of Chisso.

Second, the criteria for the diagnosis of Minamata disease, which are described in the procedure about how to fill in the uniform medical certificate, take account of decisions in past trials where the clinical picture of Minamata disease was contested. That is, the accuracy of these criteria for diagnosis has already been confirmed in court; these are criteria that lead to the appropriate relief of victims in court.

Third, the uniform medical certificate carefully selected symptoms for examination necessary and sufficient to relieve large numbers of plaintiffs swiftly and appropriately. By examining symptoms written in the certificate, doctors can diagnose each of the plaintiffs as suffering from Minamata disease, and can also understand the extent of sufferings.

We decided that we made individual certificates according to the format of this uniform medical certificate and submitted them to the court. These certificates were enough to prove each of the plaintiffs to be a Minamata disease sufferer, we thought.

(2-3) The cross-examination of Dr. Shigeru Takaoka
To prove that the above theory of the clinical picture or the uniform

medical certificate was trustworthy, we conducted the cross-examination of Dr. Shigeru Takaoka. Dr. Takaoka had treated and studied Minamata disease patients in Minamata for many years; he also took the initiative in creating the uniform medical certificate. This important cross-examination started on July 25, 2007, and, after three direct examinations and four cross-examinations, ended on July 3, 2009. Lasting as long as two years, this cross-examination turned out to be so significant as to be recorded in the history of Minamata disease trials: it revealed the latest theory of the clinical picture of Minamata disease.

First of all, Minamata disease is an unprecedented pollution-related disease that human beings experienced for the first time. The only way to grasp its true nature is to study many patients who are complaining about health problems in the coastal areas of the Shiranui Sea. The study to understand the whole picture of Minamata disease had been extremely insufficient, but the nature of Minamata disease was being revealed by groups such as the team of medical doctors of the Minamata Disease Citizens' Council. The team's representative work was the epidemiological study on Katsura Island by Dr. Tadashi Fujino, "The Clinical and Epidemiological Study on Chronic Minamata Disease."

Given such achievements or his own latest medical research findings, Dr. Takaoka argued in his testimony that superficial sensory disorders in the distal portion of all four extremities or systemic superficial sensory disorders can be highly characteristically recognized in Minamata disease patients, and that, if those who have been exposed to methyl mercury exhibit these symptoms, they can be diagnosed as suffering from Minamata disease. In response to this testimony, the national and Kumamoto prefectural governments and Chisso insisted, "basing the diagnosis on systemic sensory disorders is inconsistent with pathological findings in organs such as cerebrums." Dr. Takaoka refuted saying that pathological findings have their limitations or that not only his team's observations but also other doctors' observations confirmed the phenomenon of systemic sensory disorders, which should be taken seriously.

The uniform medical certificates that we submitted to the court were standardized in terms of the method for examination, the method to judge normality or abnormality, the criteria for diagnosis, and the format.

According to the testimony by Dr. Takaoka, the diagnosis of sensory disorders adopted the common method using a writing brush and a needle; the credibility of findings was improved because the method for examination and the method to judge abnormality were standardized, taking account of the results of studies such as the quantification of sensory testing and a study on the unpolluted area.

The national government, the defendant, argued, "the findings of sensory disorders lack objectivity," but Dr. Takaoka made a bitter counterargument, saying that determining the presence or absence of sensory disorders with a writing brush and a needle was a basic method in neurology, and that the argument put forward by the defendants was exactly equivalent to denying medicine.

The defendants also repeatedly asked whether Dr. Takaoka's view "obtain[ed] consensus in medicine," or "[was] adopted in textbooks." Dr. Takaoka answered that there was no such thing as a textbook, with clinical and epidemiological studies on Minamata disease hardly conducted, adding that the strict criteria for certification, the "1977 Certification Criteria," decided by the national government prevented many doctors from conducting clinical research to reveal widespread sufferings.

This testimony shed light on the unreasonable stance of the defendants who failed to face reality while sticking to the 1977 Certification Criteria, which trivialized the sufferings of Minamata disease.

Considering the uniform medical certificates and their underlying materials, such as interview sheets and clinical charts, Dr. Takaoka testified that all the fifty plaintiffs of the First Part "suffer[ed] from

Minamata disease."

Although the defendants insisted that the plaintiffs' illnesses were "caused by other diseases or factors," Dr. Takaoka argued that the format itself of the uniform medical certificate included enough symptoms to differentiate Minamata disease from other diseases. In addition, according to him, doctors had conducted sufficient differential diagnosis in preparing the uniform medical certificates; it was rather the defendants that were putting forward an unfounded argument about differential diagnosis.

In this way, the testimony of Dr. Takaoka proved the credibility of the uniform medical certificates. This testimony turned out to be very effective in making a rule in settlement negotiations with the defendants later. Concerning the rule for a settlement, the defendants had probably wanted to "base the judgment of relief recipients not on the uniform medical certificates but on official medical certificates issued by doctors who were selected by the defendants." But, after all, they agreed to "use the unified medical certificates and official medical certificates equally in the judgment." This was a rule based on the assumption that doctors' findings written in the unified medical certificates were credible — a rule that would not have been realized if the testimony of Dr. Takaoka had not succeeded.

That is why the cross-examination of Dr. Takaoka produced excellent results in realizing the relief of Minamata disease victims.

(2-4) The failure of the opportunist scholar Motoo Fujiki (the cross-examination on November 13, 2009)
In the No-More-Minamata Lawsuit, besides the clinical picture of Minamata disease, it was also an important point of contention whether the national and Kumamoto prefectural governments and Chisso could escape the responsibility for compensation according to stipulations with regard to extinctive prescription or the term of exclusion, which are

stipulated in Article 724 of the Civil Law Act.

The national and Kumamoto prefectural governments argued that they were not responsible for compensation because the term of exclusion had expired around a year after the trial started, on November 20, 2006 — twenty years after the symptoms of Minamata disease appeared in the plaintiffs. Chisso also insisted that the twenty-year term of exclusion had expired on September 28, 2006. Moreover, Chisso suddenly brought forward the "three-year extinctive prescription," which it had never mentioned since the First Minamata Disease Lawsuit, and rejected the responsibility for compensation on this ground.

Particularly Chisso resorted entirely to extinctive prescription and the term of exclusion, saying to the plaintiffs as follows:

> The sudden demand for compensation by the plaintiffs, who clearly changed their minds in the face of the Supreme Court decision on the Kansai Lawsuit, is (…) totally unacceptable. Some victims had demanded compensation from the defendant Chisso for many years until the 1996 comprehensive solution — presumably meaning the 1995 political solution — was reached, while the plaintiffs had almost rested on their rights, doing nothing even at the time of the comprehensive solution, and now suddenly file a lawsuit. It is extremely irrational to deal with these two groups equally in terms of prescription and exclusion. (a brief dated April 27, 2007)

These arguments were inexcusable. the national and Kumamoto prefectural governments and Chisso tried to escape their responsibility only on the ground of the passage of time even if the plaintiffs were Minamata disease patients or Minamata disease victims.

These arguments by the national and Kumamoto prefectural governments and Chisso were based on the interpretation of the term of exclusion that the 2004 Supreme Court decision on the Kansai Lawsuit had accepted to a certain extent. That is, this decision judged that, because of the term of exclusion, the national and Kumamoto prefectural governments were not responsible for compensating plaintiffs who had moved to distant places such as Kansai, "if they did not apply for certification within twenty-four years after moving," even if the plaintiffs were Minamata disease victims.

This judgment was utterly unfair, ignoring the fact that victims could not come forward as Minamata disease sufferers because of discrimination or prejudice even if they did have its symptoms. However, because this judgment was indeed presented in the decision, and, in court, many judges tend to follow precedents established by the Supreme Court, we expected that the term of exclusion would become an important legal point of contention also in the No-More-Minamata Lawsuit.

To strike back the cross-examination of Dr. Shigeru Takaoka, the national and Kumamoto prefectural governments arranged the cross-examination of the witness Motoo Fujiki. The witness Fujiki was originally a researcher in the measurement of minuscule quantities of mercury. In the No-More-Minamata Lawsuit, he testified, "there is no pollution by methyl mercury enough to cause Minamata disease after 1969, when the production of acetaldehyde stopped," relying on the findings of studies on the level of mercury contained in fish and shellfish in Minamata Bay, the hair of residents, or the navel strings of newborns of residents. In fact, the witness Fujiki had consistently presented reasons to reject the responsibility of the national and Kumamoto prefectural governments as a witness of the national government since the so-called Third Minamata Disease Lawsuit: "given scientific knowledge around 1955, the national and Kumamoto prefectural governments don't have to take responsibility for the spread of the sufferings of Minamata disease," he had testified.

By arguing in the No-More-Minamata Lawsuit that there had been no pollution enough to cause Minamata disease after 1969, his testimony supported the view that the twenty-year term of exclusion had expired for all the plaintiffs.

Although the witness Fujiki testified, "there is no pollution enough to cause Minamata disease after 1969," he could not squarely refute doctors saying that the symptoms of Minamata disease could also be recognized among residents who were born after 1969.

Because the No-More-Minamata Lawsuit was concluded with a victorious out-of-court settlement, the court did not judge the view of the witness Fujiki. His testimony, however, was substantially entirely discarded: no plaintiff was rejected the settlement on the ground of the passage of time in the settlement in 2011; and the plaintiffs who were born after 1969 were included in the settlement, although partly.

Using other cases of lawsuits, the No-More-Minamata defense team held a symposium on extinctive prescription and the term of exclusion. Supported by researchers and lawyers, the team also submitted a brief saying that the argument based on prescription and exclusion was itself equivalent to the abuse of rights, given the stance of the offenders who had prevented the cause of Minamata disease from being revealed and hidden sufferings. The brief also advocated that all Minamata disease victims should be compensated by reckoning prescription and exclusion from the time of diagnosis or certification.

But in overcoming the point of contention about prescription and exclusion, the most essential was "to disclose that there [were] still many neglected Minamata disease victims." Therefore, we could overcome the arguments related to prescription and exclusion made by the national and prefectural governments and Chisso because we increased the number of plaintiffs ultimately to about 3,000; we maintained the firm solidarity of the plaintiff group; in unison with the team of medical doctors and supporters, we conducted the campaign to uncover Minamata disease victims; and particularly because we succeeded in organizing medical examinations of 1,044 residents in total in the coastal areas of the Shiranui Sea — the above-mentioned Mass Medical Examinations.

3. Nationwide Campaigns

(1) Minamata disease is not yet over: the Minamata Caravan across Japan

Needless to say, our battle was launched by victims who were stimulated by the 2004 Supreme Court decision on the Kansai Lawsuit. However, because the 1995 political solution relieved many Minamata disease victims, it was generally understood across the country that Minamata disease had been settled. Our first challenge was to change such public sentiment and to make the public aware of the fact that many Minamata disease victims were still left neglected, and the necessity to relieve them. So we carried on the Minamata Caravan across Japan over about two months from May 16, 2008, traveling from Kumamoto to Hokkaido under the slogan, "Minamata disease is not yet over."

The day of the departure ceremony of the caravan was also the day when the 13th oral proceedings in the No-More-Minamata Lawsuit took place, where the cross-examination of Dr. Shigeru Takaoka, who had diagnosed the large majority of the plaintiffs, was accepted — the day when the trial took a big step forward. Not only the plaintiff group and defense team but also nurses from the Kumamoto Prefecture Liaison Council to Support Minamata Disease Battles joined in the caravan, so that they could treat the plaintiffs who joined in the caravan departing from the Kumamoto District Court when their condition got worse.

Visiting Fukuoka Prefecture on May 18, 2008, the first part of the caravan subsequently went to Hiroshima, Okayama, Hyogo, Osaka, Kyoto, Aichi, and Kanagawa Prefectures, eight prefectures in total; it visited prefectural offices, asked organizations for support, and conducted advertising campaigns on the streets. The participating plaintiffs concretely explained "sensory disorders," the symptom of Minamata disease that was not recognized apparently. The voices of victims

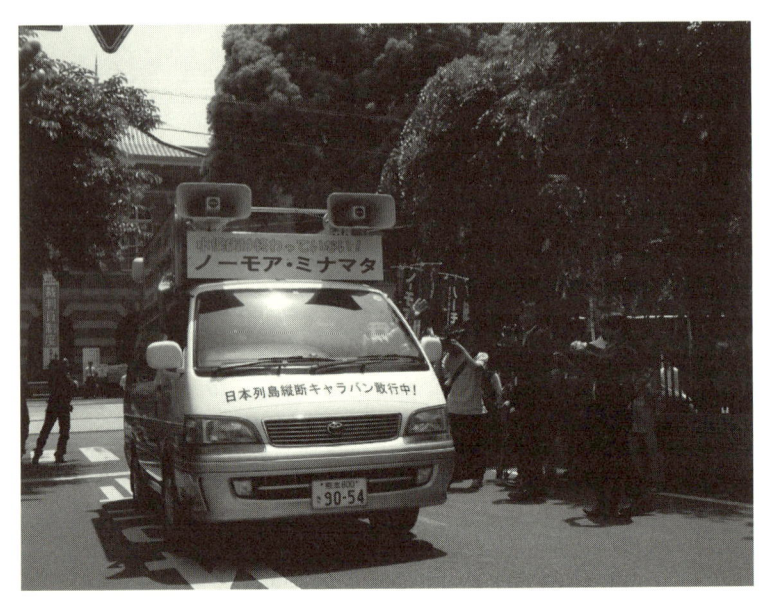

Photo 11. Departure ceremony of the Minamata Caravan
Photo: Hideo Kitaoka

themselves shocked those who had not known Minamata disease; they deeply understood that Minamata disease victims were still suffering even fifty years after the disease was officially recognized. The media covered the caravan in each place; we were surprised at their great interest in our campaign. After the Nationwide General Action of Pollution Victims on June 2 and 3, 2008, we started the latter half of the caravan from June 12. In the latter half, after making a thorough appeal in Tokyo, we went to ten prefectures — Chiba, Saitama, Ibaragi, Tochigi, Gunma, Niigata, Fukushima, Yamagata, Iwate, and Aomori — and entered Hokkaido.

The reason why we headed for Hokkaido was that the Toyako Summit was to be held there in July 2008; we wanted to bring the world's attention to the fact that there was a pollution issue unresolved over more than fifty years in Japan, the chair country for the summit. As a matter of

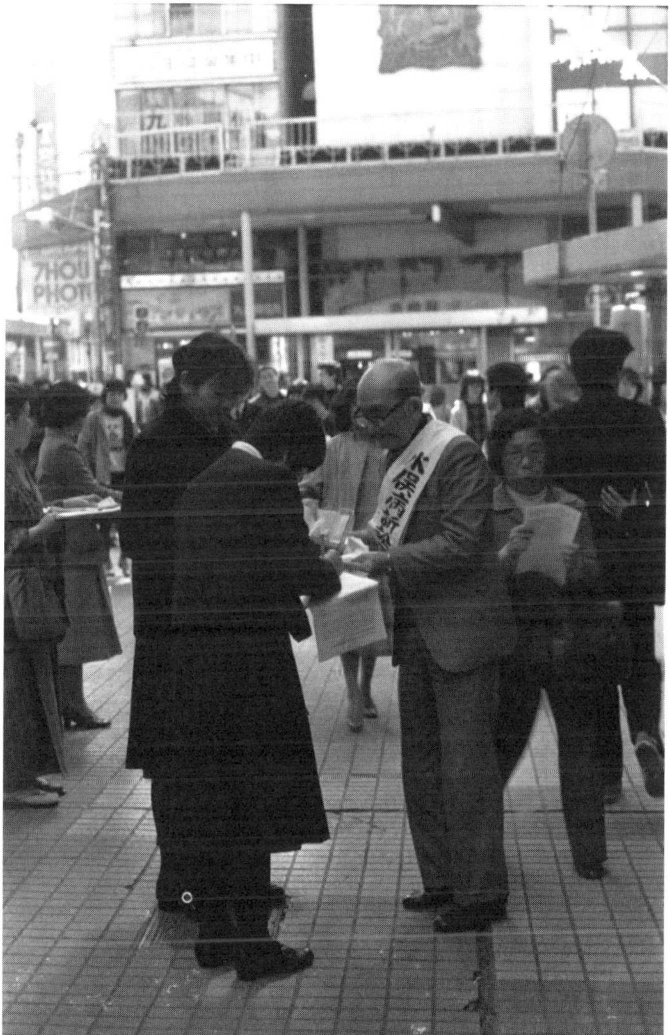

Photo 12. Street campaign
On the streets, some appealed for support for Minamata disease victims while some signed heartily. Photo: Hideo Kitaoka

course, we were not allowed to enter the venue of the summit, but kept the caravan continuous to Hokkaido, where we participated in an international symposium in Sapporo or joined in a talk session in Odori Park. In Hokkaido, far from Kumamoto, we stressed, "Minamata disease is not over," concluding the caravan of about one and a half months with success. The caravan was better known in the latter half, with the media covering it widely. What the caravan had achieved was not only the nationwide support; all the plaintiffs joining in the caravan also gained confidence because they really understood that it could arouse sympathy and great support among people to talk about the sufferings of Minamata disease — something that they had not been able to do so far. Having grown up as a movement with supporters across the country, we kept carrying on active campaigns such as advertising campaigns in Minamata and attempts to increase plaintiffs.

With regard to nationwide campaigns, we had participated in the Nationwide General Action of Pollution Victims every year, where victims' groups of pollution or drug-induced diseases gathered from all over the country and conducted negotiations with ministries and agencies concerned or offending companies, rallies, demonstrations on the streets, advertising campaigns, and so on. Minamata disease issues had come to be treated as a central topic in the Nationwide General Action. The participation in the action strengthened solidarity with victims of pollution or drug-induced diseases like us, providing a firm foothold for nationwide campaigns.

(2) Refusing to end with the Law Concerning Special Measures

The Law Concerning Special Measures for the Relief of Minamata Disease Victims and the Settlement of Minamata Disease Issues was enacted on July 8, 2009. A campaign to prevent this law from being enacted also helped our battle to make enormous progress.

The Law Concerning Special Measures was proposed in exchange for relief measures prepared by the Government Parties' Project Team for Minamata Disease Issues; Chisso, who ought to make lump-sum payments, rejected those relief measures, saying, "these don't realize a final solution," because the Association "SHIRANUI" flatly turned down those measures. Although the law nominally advocated the relief of Minamata disease victims, the planned relief was extremely insufficient; the law was substantially intended to divide the offending company Chisso. Extremely insufficient, because this law was based on a scheme in which the national government, whose responsibility for Minamata disease had been established, selected victims eligible for relief. Such a scheme would necessarily lead to abandoning large numbers of victims. Some of victims' groups welcomed this law, but we could not accept this, regarding this as a law that rather relieved offenders and abandoned victims while just nominally relieving victims.

We launched a campaign to prevent the law from being enacted in March 2009, when the law surfaced as a proposal by the government's parties. First of all, to emphasize how unacceptable it was to divide Chisso, we organized an emergency symposium on March 4 the same year, where Masafumi Yokemoto, associate professor at Tokyo Keizai University, lectured on the scheme — the framework, aim, and implication — of the division in plain language.

On March 13 the same year, when the cross-examination of Dr. Takaoka was conducted, to further strengthen the solidarity of the plaintiff group, we organized an "emergency meeting to protest against having presented the Law Concerning Special Measures to the Diet" during the lunch hour in the cross-examination. At this meeting, we confirmed that we did not accept a solution based on the law, continuing the trial, and that we informed members of the Diet of our view.

From around this time, we frequently went to Tokyo, where we urged members of the Diet to resolve Minamata disease issues fairly. On June 2, we held an emergency meeting within the Diet Building, where many members of the Diet from nongovernment parties participated and promised solidarity with us. But the Democratic Party, a nongovernment party in those days, dismissed the chair of the "Democratic Party's Minamata Disease Working Team," a member of the House of Councilors from the Kumamoto electoral district, and co-opted him into the party executive, so that the party aimed for an agreement with the Liberal Democratic Party. With such a move of the Democratic Party, the enactment of the Law Concerning Special Measures became more of a real possibility.

To highlight the unfairness of the law without giving up to the last ditch, we staged a sit-in in front of the Diet Building from June 25. We also petitioned, among others, members of the Diet who belonged to the Committee on the Environment, while continuing an advertising campaign in front of the Diet Building. Various people expressed support for our campaign. Particularly it brought public attention to the unfairness of the law that Kunio Yanagida and Takeko Kato expressed opposition to the law; both of them were members of the Council on Minamata Disease Issues, which was formed by the Minister of the Environment in 2005.

Victims' groups opposing the law also cooperated. We cooperated with the Niigata Minamata Disease Agano Victim's Group for this campaign, and later formed with it the No More Minamata Disease National Liaison Council of Victims and Defense Teams, fighting together until a settlement was reached. The circle of support for us went on widening noticeably. Thanks to the sit-in staged day after day, many people rallied around us: members of the Diet, the executives of support groups, or victims of other pollution. The cooperation cultivated during this campaign must have greatly contributed toward widening the circle of support in Tokyo and filing a lawsuit in Tokyo later.

On July 2, 2009, despite our thorough opposition, the Liberal Democratic Party, New Komeito, and Democratic Party reached an agreement on the Law Concerning Special Measures, which was enacted after the House of Representatives and the House of Councilors passed it on July 3 and 8, respectively. We were furious about the enactment of the law, but, ironically, settling Minamata disease issues became urgent for the national government because Minamata disease issues were reported across the country thanks to the enactment of the law, attracting public attention. In addition, as a result of the campaign to block the enactment of the law and committed persuasion by members of the Diet who belonged to the Democratic Party's Minamata Disease Working Team, the content of the law became more effective in relieving victims.

(3) The battle after the enactment of the Law Concerning Special Measures

In the campaign against the Law Concerning Special Measures, we learned that fighting to the last ditch without giving up could lead to a great success. The law only stipulated the framework for the relief of Minamata disease victims; the substance of the relief was not yet decided at all. We needed to make the relief as helpful as possible, for victims who had not been involved in the trial as well. To realize a higher level of the relief, we kept going to Tokyo even after the law was enacted, and published newsletters introducing our view, appealing to members of the Diet. We continued our effort to increase plaintiffs, and also realized a lawsuit in the capital, Tokyo.

One of the achievements of these efforts was certainly the 2011 victorious settlement.

Our battle, however, is not over with this. Under the slogan, the "relief of all Minamata disease victims," we will keep fighting as long as there are neglected victims. And we have to promulgate the lessons of Minamata disease not only domestically but also globally.

Chapter 3
The Content and Achievements of the 2011 Victorious Settlement

1. Until the Basic Agreement based on the Opinion on Settlement

After the Law Concerning Special Measures was enacted on July 8, 2009, we decided to demand a swift out-of-court settlement based on legal negotiations from the national and prefectural governments and Chisso, while proving, "it is after all the judicature that relieves all Minamata disease victims."

Also in the No-More-Minamata Lawsuit, the defendants had persistently interpreted the clinical picture of Minamata disease narrowly, saying, "we don't recognize victims as suffering from Minamata disease unless they exhibit multiple symptoms other than sensory disorders," or "symptoms other than sensory disorders in the distal portion of all four extremities cannot be regarded as symptoms characteristic of Minamata disease." Given the cross-examination of Dr Shigeru Takaoka, however, the Law Concerning Special Measures could not but recognize victims only with sensory disorders as suffering from Minamata disease or also victims with systemic sensory disorders as such.

Or the defendants had demanded limitations based on extinctive prescription and the term of exclusion, saying, "the plaintiffs filed the lawsuit too late." Faced with the increasing number of victims, however, the law could not impose limitations based on the term.

Thus the two main points of contention that the defendants had put forward in the lawsuit were substantially resolved by the enactment of the law. So the plaintiff group filed an additional lawsuit with sixty-nine plaintiffs on July 31 the same year. On August 9 the same year, it organized a rally with 1,200 participants and resolved to fight under the slogan, "the defendants should now come to the negotiating table for a swift out-of-court settlement based on legal negotiations."

In Minamata City on August 23 the same year, the "No More Minamata Disease National Liaison Council of Victims and Defense Teams" (the No More Council) was formed by the plaintiff groups and defense teams in Kumamoto, the Kinki Region, and Niigata, and the defense team in Tokyo. Later, the plaintiff group in Tokyo also joined it. The No More Council played an important role not only in relieving hidden victims across the country, but also in coordinating settlement negotiations later.

On September 20 and 21 the same year, medical examinations of about 1,000 residents were conducted at seventeen venues in the coastal areas of the Shiranui Sea. The chair for this event was Masazumi Harada. Its details were already mentioned. The results of these examinations revealed that there were many unnoticed victims in areas or generations where governments had assumed "there [were] no Minamata disease victims"; the defendants were shocked at the results.

And in November the same year, the national government was finally forced to start prior consultation with the plaintiff group aiming for a judicial settlement. In the consultation, we mainly discussed the content of compensation or the method to judge victims, identifying issues involved. On January 22, 2010, the Kumamoto District Court (Chief Justice Ryosuke Takahashi) issued a recommendation for settlement to both parties, who immediately entered into settlement negotiations. In the negotiations, both parties expressed to the court their wishes concerning not only the content of compensation or the method to judge victims but also areas or ages eligible for relief.

On the other hand, twelve victims living in the Kinki Region filed a lawsuit in the Osaka District Court on February 27, 2009; twenty-three victims living in the Kanto Region, in the Tokyo District Court on February 23, 2010 — immediately after the settlement negotiations started in the Kumamoto District Court. These lawsuits in the Kinki and Kanto Regions not only accelerated the settlement negotiations but also forced the national government to recognize the necessity to relieve victims who had moved outside Kumamoto Prefecture.

On March 15, 2010, after three settlement negotiations, the Kumamoto District Court presented its opinion on settlement. Forming the main points of the settlement mentioned below, this opinion incorporated wishes of the plaintiffs asking for wide-ranging relief: it stipulated relief consisting of three major payments — lump-sum payments, medical expenses, and medical allowances; the method to judge victims in a third-party committee; or the method to judge victims including the plaintiffs living outside existing eligible areas. The plaintiff group immediately organized meetings in twenty-nine areas, where a total of more than 1,000 plaintiffs participated and discussed the opinion. Then, on March 28 the same year, it organized a general meeting with 1,050 participants at Minamata City General Gymnasium, where it was decided to accept the opinion by an overwhelming majority. Because the defendants had also accepted the opinion, a basic agreement for settlement was signed in the Kumamoto District Court on March 29 the same year.

2. From Judging Victims to Reaching the Settlement

The plaintiff group explained to all the plaintiffs about the significance of the third-party diagnosis or its following procedures. As a result of negotiations, the plaintiffs who died before the third-party diagnosis could also be relieved, if they had undergone official medical examinations while in life, by using the results.

For the plaintiffs living outside existing eligible areas, including those in Amakusa except for Goshoura, we made or collected materials proving that they had eaten large amounts of fish from around Minamata Bay.

After lawyers interviewed each of the plaintiffs and recorded the result according to the format of a deposition, officials of the Kumamoto and Kagoshima prefectural governments interviewed the plaintiff in the presence of lawyers.

The third-party committee consisted of five members: chair Masazumi Yoshii (the former mayor of Minamata City), two doctors nominated by the plaintiffs, and two doctors nominated by the defendants. The committee engaged in an intense and impartial discussion every time referring to the results of diagnosis or epidemiological materials. Given judgments made by the committee, we organized meetings in thirty areas, where a total of more than 1,700 plaintiffs participated and discussed whether we should accept the settlement. On March 21, 2011, we held a general meeting with 1,512 participants at Ashikita Sky Dome; we decided to sign the settlement by an overwhelming majority. Subsequently, settlements were reached in the Tokyo District Court on March 24, in the Kumamoto District Court on March 25, and in the Osaka District Court on March 28.

3. The Content of the Settlement

The compensation comprises three major payments: 1) medical expenses, 2) medical allowances, and 3) lump-sum payments.

Eligible victims do not have to pay medical expenses any more because the copayment is covered by the national and prefectural governments. They can get treatment without anxiety throughout their

The Content and Achievements of the 2011 Victorious Settlement

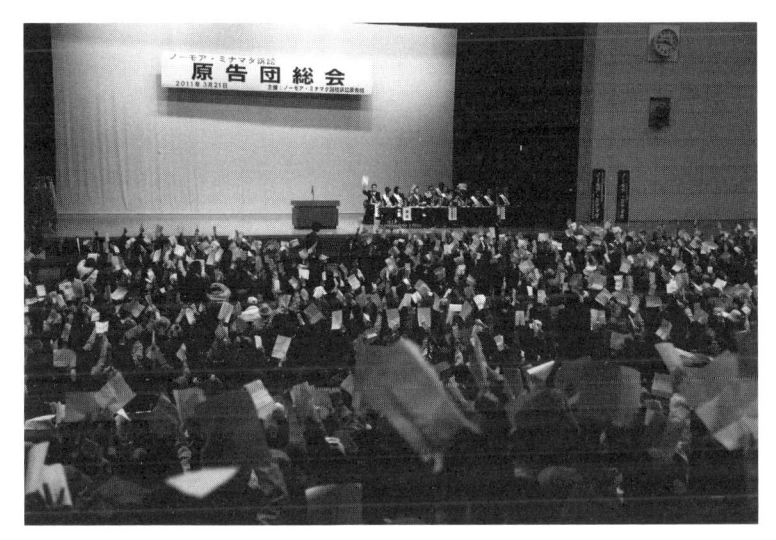

Photo 13. General meeting of plaintiffs on March 21, 2011
Photo: Hideo Kitaoka

lives.

The medical allowances per month are 17,000 yen for an inpatient, 15,900 yen for an outpatient of 70 years old and over, and 12,900 yen for an outpatient under 70 years old. These are also ample compensation as lifetime allowances.

The lump-sum payments were 3,450 million yen for groups — including payments for the Kinki Region and Tokyo — as well as 2.1 million yen for individuals. These were short of the levels stipulated by the 2004 Supreme Court decision on the Kansai Lawsuit. But these can be still regarded as excellent results of the battle of the plaintiff group, considering that three major payments including medical expenses and medical allowances are offered, and that these were achieved after a relatively short period of time, five and a half years after the lawsuit was filed.

Arousing criticism, the director of the Environmental Health

Department of the Ministry of the Environment uttered following wild words as if the plaintiffs were "bogus patients":
> We can't see if examinees are lying.
>
> People in the coastal areas of the Shiranui Sea tend to quickly link poor physical condition with Minamata disease.
>
> Surveys biased by money don't reveal what medical causes are.

Therefore, it was also significant for the plaintiffs to have achieved the settlement after the defendants admitted that the plaintiffs suffered from Minamata disease.

The basic agreement stated that "the defendants [should] examine how to actually express their responsibility and apology." As a result, then Prime Minister Yukio Hatoyama attended the Minamata Disease Victims Memorial Service as the first prime minister to attend the service, saying, "I admit the responsibility for having failed to prevent the sufferings of Minamata disease from spreading, and once again apologize from the bottom of my heart," while the Kumamoto prefectural governor also apologized.

In addition, the settlement stipulated as follows:
> To objectively understand the relationship between methyl mercury and its effects on health, the national government shall conduct a study using latest medical knowledge, enlisting the cooperation and participation of those concerned in the local community including the plaintiffs. It shall try to start the development of methods for the study without delay.

This stipulation gives the Association "SHIRANUI," which strives for the "relief of all Minamata disease victims," a foothold toward realizing medical examinations of residents in the coastal areas of the Shiranui Sea.

4. The Significance of the Judicial Settlement

Apart from the payments, this settlement can be regarded as significant in the following four respects.

First, this settlement was achieved because we forced the national government to come to the judicial negotiating table for the first time in the history of Minamata disease trials over forty years, and forced it to search for solutions with the plaintiffs. The 2004 Supreme Court decision on the Kansai Lawsuit established the legal responsibility of the national and Kumamoto prefectural governments for the spread of Minamata disease, substantially rejecting the strict criteria for certification used by the national government. Faced with this decision, the fifty plaintiffs filed the No-More-Minamata Lawsuit in the Kumamoto District Court in 2005; they proposed, "negotiations in court should decide a rule — a judicial relief scheme — that relieves large numbers of victims quickly." If there had been only fifty victims eligible for compensation for Minamata disease, it might have been possible for all the plaintiffs to pursue a ruling. However, by 2005, when the First Part of the plaintiffs filed a lawsuit, more than 1,000 victims had already submitted applications for certification to the Kumamoto and Kagoshima prefectural governments; it was clear that there were still many hidden victims who had not yet come forward. To relieve thousands or tens of thousands of victims quickly, therefore, it was necessary and possible to reach an out-of-court settlement with the national and Kumamoto prefectural governments and Chisso in line with the 2004 Supreme Court decision on the Kansai Lawsuit, we supposed, and proposed establishing a judicial relief scheme.

In response to our proposal, the Minister of the Environment in those days when the First Part of the lawsuit was filed in 2005 bluntly said, "we won't seek a settlement with the plaintiffs." Faced with the increasing number of plaintiffs even after the Law Concerning Special Measures was enacted in 2009, however, the national government had to switch its policy, saying, "we will strive for a judicial settlement with the plaintiffs." And, before deciding the specifics of the law, the government repeatedly negotiated with the plaintiff group to decide a rule for settlement. As long as a judicial settlement was strived for, convincing the plaintiff group of the settlement was essential, which led to utterly different results than results one-sided judgments based on the Law Concerning Special Measures would have brought about. Consequently, we were able to establish a rule stipulating that a third-party committee should judge victims — a rule to relieve large numbers of plaintiffs swiftly and fairly. Of 2,992 plaintiffs including those in the Kinki Region and Tokyo, 2,772 plaintiffs (92.6%) were judged to be eligible for a lump-sum payment; combined with 22 plaintiffs who were eligible only for medical expenses, 93.3% of the plaintiffs were relieved.

Second, this settlement was epoch-making in that it discarded the selection of victims by governments alone, introducing a "third-party committee." So far, the national government had consistently adhered to the theory of the foundation of governance, insisting, "governments — doctors selected by governments — decide 'who victims are'." The plaintiff group criticized this theory, saying, "it is inappropriate for the national government, which was condemned as an offender in the Supreme Court decision, to decide 'who victims are'." And we conducted the cross-examination of Dr. Shigeru Takaoka, proving the credibility of the "uniform medical certificates" made by the team of doctors of the Citizens' Council. As a consequence, the opinion on settlement presented by the Kumamoto District Court adopted the method to judge victims based on the "third-party committee," half of whose members were to be selected by the plaintiff group. The opinion also regarded the "uniform medical certificates" made by the team of doctors of the Citizens' Council as equal to the third-party (official) medical certificates in judging victims. In other words, we broke through governments' monopoly of the authority to judge "who [were] Minamata disease victims."

Also in terms of the clinical picture, which the national government had tried to interpret narrowly, the settlement was effective in increasing eligible victims, recognizing systemic sensory disorders as a symptom of Minamata disease, for example. These achievements must have an enormous impact on the certification of other pollution victims and victims of drug-induced diseases.

Third, the settlement significantly expanded the area eligible for relief: even in areas that had not been eligible for relief so far, such as Amakusa, about 70% of applicants were certified. So far, governments had demarcated the area eligible for relief according to municipal boundaries and rejected relief for those living outside the area, regarding them as not exposed to methyl mercury. However, making depositions concerning the consumption of fish and shellfish, standing by during interviews by the prefectural governments, and negotiating a settlement persistently, we forced governments to admit that there were many victims in areas where governments had insisted, "there are no Minamata disease victims." This achievement greatly contributed toward providing relief based on the Law Concerning Special Measures in those areas. Considering the time of exposure, relief had been limited to those who were born by the end of 1968. We extended this time until November 30, 1969, while those who were born after this date were also to be relieved under certain conditions. Having broken through such demarcation based on areas and ages is a great step toward the "relief of all victims."

Fourth, the settlement was also epoch-making in realizing relief without prescription and exclusion. Chisso argued that the plaintiffs' right to demand compensation had lapsed because of prescription, telling them, "those who rest on the rights are not eligible for protection." The national and Kumamoto prefectural governments also insisted that the plaintiffs' claim was not accepted according to the term of exclusion, because they had contracted Minamata disease more than twenty years before. Indeed, in some trials related to pneumoconiosis (work-related illness) or hepatitis (drug-induced disease), plaintiffs' claim is limited because of the term of exclusion. In the No-More-Minamata Lawsuit, however, adopting the principle that "there is no prescription for pollution," we argued in and outside court, "it is essentially against fair and equitable principles and unacceptable that Chisso, the offending company, insists on extinctive prescription." Concerning the term of exclusion put forward by the national and prefectural governments, we emphasized, "how difficult it was for victims to come forward as Minamata disease sufferers immediately after they contracted the disease, given difficulty in diagnosing the disease and deep-rooted discrimination and prejudice." In the face of large numbers of victims, the national government could not stipulate the term of exclusion in the Law Concerning Special Measures, nor could it insist on discrimination based on the term of exclusion in the No-More-Minamata Lawsuit.

These four achievements are the fruits of the battle of the No-More-Minamata Lawsuit.

Conclusion
Remaining Minamata Disease Issues

On July 31, 2012, the Ministry of the Environment terminated the acceptance of application for relief measures based on the Law Concerning Special Measures for the Relief of Minamata Disease Victims and the Settlement of Minamata Disease Issues. By this date, a total of 65,151 victims had applied. Although governments do not reveal how they had addressed those applications, Chisso had made a lump-sum payment of 2.1 million yen per person to 27,770 victims among those who are eligible for the relief based on the law, according to the March 2013 consolidated accounts of Chisso and other documents. The way to handle an objection, however, is different depending on governments: the ministry and Kumamoto and Kagoshima prefectural governments insist that victims who were not relieved by the law cannot raise an objection; the Niigata prefectural government accepts an objection from the victims.

In addition, concerning the deadline for application, it is pointed out that the national and prefectural governments have made it impossible for the following victims to apply.

First, when the contamination was serious, peddlers carried the contaminated fish to mountainous areas, where victims have not been uncovered well.

Second, victims have not been uncovered well who live outside areas eligible for the relief in Kumamoto and Kagoshima Prefectures: those living in Amakusa, Kumamoto Prefecture, and those living in inland areas of Kagoshima Prefecture.

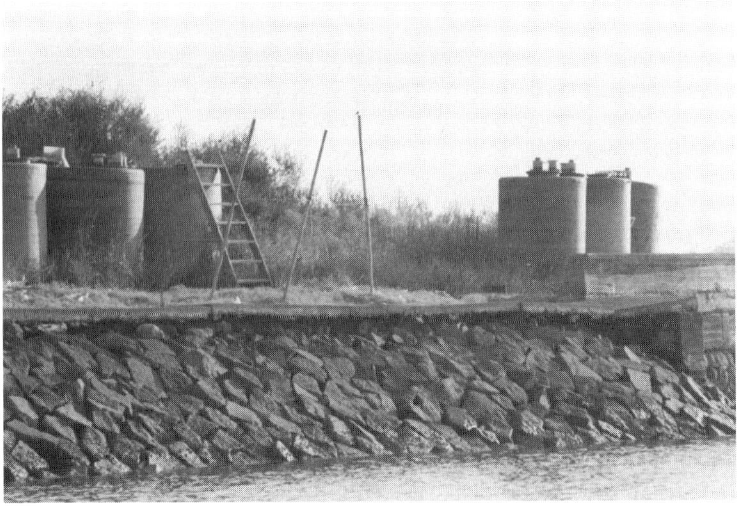

Photo 14. Dumpsters for contaminated fish
Contaminated fish from Minamata Bay were collected and dumped in tanks. Photo: Hideo Kitaoka

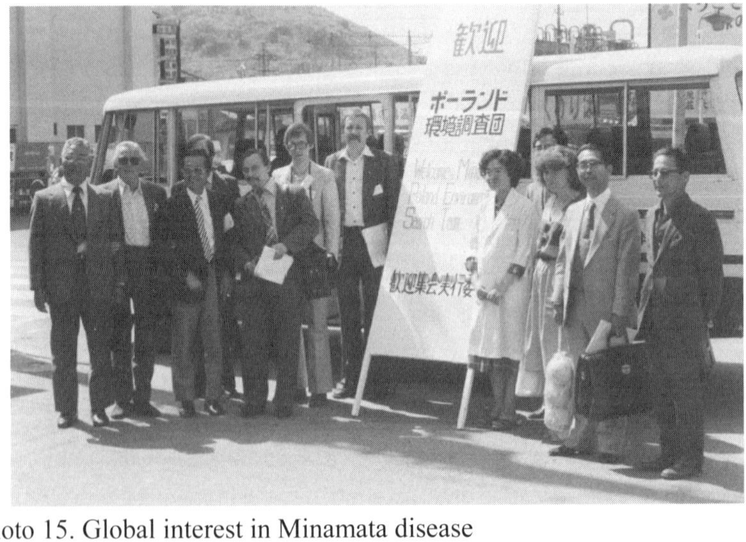

Photo 15. Global interest in Minamata disease
Research groups from across the world were determined not to allow the same fault to be committed again in other countries. Photo: Hideo Kitaoka

Third, the law relieves victims who were born by December 1968, by when they are supposed to have contracted Minamata disease, but does not relieve those who were born after that. The judicial settlement reached in March 2011, however, does relieve those subject to this limitation and the second limitation. In the future, it is necessary to remove the limitation by the law.

Fourth, for example, in Tsunagi Town, the heavily polluted area, half of its residents have left the town since the time when the contamination was serious, moving to cities. They have not been investigated.

In January 2011, Chisso established JNC Inc. in accordance with the law; it transferred all its businesses to JNC in April the same year. But the Supreme Court decision on October 15, 2004, recognized the responsibility of the national and Kumamoto prefectural governments to compensate victims only with sensory disorders. Therefore, as long as Minamata disease victims only with sensory disorders are not relieved, all Minamata disease victims are not relieved.

Moreover, the Supreme Court handed down a decision on April 16, 2013, that administratively certified victims only with sensory disorders as suffering from Minamata disease. Given this decision, victims only with sensory disorders can now be administratively certified as suffering from Minamata disease in court; they can also bring a civil suit for damages.

On June 20, 2013, forty-eight plaintiffs filed a lawsuit claiming compensation for Minamata disease against the national or Kumamoto prefectural government in the Kumamoto District Court.

It was on May 1, 1956, that the national government officially recognized Minamata disease. Fifty-seven years after the date, a lawsuit over Minamata disease still continues. This battle would continue until the last victim is relieved.

"Pollution starts with damage and ends with damage," it is said; Minamata disease issues are not yet settled either.

Japanese Version

ノーモア・ミナマタ
司法による解決のみち

水俣病不知火患者会、ノーモア・ミナマタ国賠等訴訟弁護団、
ノーモア・ミナマタ編集委員会　編

目　次

まえがき　　　　　　　　　　　　　　　　　　　　　　78
執筆者紹介　　　　　　　　　　　　　　　　　　　　　79

はじめに：近・現代日本社会における司法の役割　　　81
　　　猪飼隆明

1．水俣病の歴史　　　　　　　　　　　　　　　　　91

2．「ノーモア・ミナマタ国家賠償等訴訟」たたかいの記録　　101

3．2011年勝利和解の内容と成果　　　　　　　　　119

むすび：水俣病問題の今後　　　　　　　　　　　　127

まえがき

　水俣病は、人の産業活動が引き起こした極めて悲惨で深刻な人体被害であることから、公害の原点といわれています。
　水俣病は、熊本県水俣市に所在するチッソ水俣工場の廃水中に含まれていたメチル水銀により汚染された魚介類を多食することにより発症する公害病です。1956年5月1日に公式に確認されました。
　チッソは、水俣病の発生を認識していながら、無処理で廃水を不知火海に垂れ流し続けていました。国、熊本県は、水俣病の発生・拡大を防止できたのに、経済成長を優先し、十分な防止策を取りませんでした。その結果、多くの者が被害を受けたのです。
　水俣病は、狂死という重篤な人体被害から感覚障害のみという比較的軽症なものまで症状は多様ですが、病像は未だ解明し尽くされていません。また、濃厚汚染時に不知火海沿岸地域には約20万人の住民が居住しており、多くの者が汚染された魚介類を多食していたことは確実ですが、被害者数は判明していません。行政が全般的な実態調査を怠っているからです。
　水俣病被害者は、被害を否定する加害企業と行政を相手に、半世紀以上にわたって、補償を求めたたかいを続けています。
　被害者が勝訴した最高裁判所判決（2004年10月）、被害者救済のための特別措置法成立（2009年7月）後も、未だ補償を受けていない被害者のたたかいは続いています。2013年6月20日、特別措置法による補償を拒否された48名の被害者が、新たな訴訟を提起しました。被害者のたたかいは、現在も進行中なのです。
　水俣病が極めて複雑で異常な経過を辿ったのは、加害企業と行政が、公害防止と実態調査を怠ったり、被害を矮小化し続けたためです。このような過ちは、負の教訓として、世界の公害防止、被害者補償に生かされなければならないと考えます。
　この本が、少しでも役立てば、幸いです。

園田昭人（弁護士）

執筆者紹介

猪飼隆明

　大阪大学名誉教授。歴史家。幕末・維新以降の政治史・思想史・社会運動史を研究。主な著書に、『西郷隆盛』（岩波新書）、『西南戦争—戦争の大義と動員される民衆』（吉川弘文館）、『ハンナリデルと回春病院』（熊本出版文化協会）、『熊本の明治秘史』（熊本日日新聞社）などがあり、水俣病問題については、「水俣病問題成立の前提」、「国策をバックにしたチッソの企業活動」などの論考を発表、またノーモア水俣環境賞の審査委員長をつとめた。

北岡秀郎

　1943年熊本市生まれ。高校教師の後、1971年から水俣病訴訟弁護団事務局員。1975年から1996年まで月刊「みなまた」を発行し水俣病問題の発信を続ける。水俣病闘争支援熊本県連絡会議事務局長、ハンセン病国賠訴訟支援全国連事務局長、川辺川利水訴訟支援連事務局長等を歴任。水俣病問題、ハンセン病問題、川辺川ダム問題、原爆被爆者訴訟、原発事故等について刊行物で情報発信を続けている

板井優

　弁護士。水俣病訴訟弁護団事務局長として、水俣市にて8年6ヶ月間弁護士事務所を開き水俣病問題の解決に奔走し、環境を破壊する川辺川ダム建設計画を事実上中止させ、ハンセン病国賠訴訟西日本弁護団事務局長をつとめる。全国公害弁護団連絡会議の事務局長、幹事長、代表委員を歴任して公害問題に取り組む。「原発なくそう！九州玄海訴訟」弁護団共同代表として、原発の廃炉を求めるたたかいに従事している。

はじめに

近・現代日本社会における司法の役割

猪飼隆明

　本書は、一企業が、国策のあとおしを受けて展開した生産活動が、地域住民や労働者に「水俣病」というきわめて深刻な被害をもたらした事実を明らかにし、被害者の救済のための、司法を中心とした、広汎かつ息の長いたたかいの姿を描こうとするものである。わたしたちが、この司法の場をたたかいの場としてきたことの意味と意義を明らかにするために、日本における、とくに明治維新以降の近代社会において司法がいかなる位置にあったのか、第二次世界大戦後、それはどのように変化し今に至っているのか、このことに触れておくことにしたい。

1）近代日本の司法制度

　近代日本の司法制度は、1868年閏4月21日に公布された「政体書」（Constitutionの邦訳）において、権力は太政官に集中していながら、近代的法制度にならって、行政・司法・立法の三権の「分立」を規定し、大坂・兵庫・長崎・京都・横浜・函館に裁判所を設置したことに始まるが、この裁判所は地方行政機関と同義であって、独立した司法機関ではなかった。これは、廃藩置県直後の1871年7月9日に司法省が設立され、司法省裁判所・府県裁判所・区裁判所が設置されて以降もこの地方行政機関的性格は引き継がれたといえる。
　そうした性格をいくぶんでも克服して近代日本司法制度体系化の第一歩となったのは、1875年4月1日に大審院が設置され、裁判権が司法卿からここに移ってからである。すなわち、この時、大審院

―上等裁判所（東京・大阪・長崎・福島〈のち宮城〉）―府県裁判所（翌年地方裁判所に）の序列がつくられ、大審院諸裁判所職制章程・控訴上告手続・裁判事務心得がつくられたのである。

　その後、自由民権運動の高揚に対抗して政府は、1880年7月17日に刑法・治罪法を公布した。この刑法は罪刑法定主義をとり、身分による刑罰の相違を廃し、いっぽう罪を重罪・軽罪・違警罪にわけた。また治罪法によって、刑事裁判手続、裁判所の種類・構成等を規定し、それぞれの罪ごとに、始審裁判所から大審院にいたる控訴・上告のシステムがつくられた。

　このように、根本法たる憲法の制定に先立って司法制度の基礎が、国民の運動との対抗の中でつくられたのである。そして、裁判所官制が制定されて、裁判官・検察官の登用、任用資格、裁判官の身分保障、司法行政の監督の系列がつくられるのは1886年5月のことであり、大日本帝国憲法の発布をうけて、かつ1890年の帝国議会の開会を前に、裁判所構成法、民事訴訟法、刑事訴訟法が相次いで制定されるのである。1893年3月公布された弁護士法については後に触れる。

2）弁護士制度時代

（1）代言人制度時代

　さて、司法の場と私法の外（地域や社会）とを結びつける役割を演じるのが弁護士であるが、いかなる制度的特徴をもっていたか。弁護士は当初は「代言人」と呼ばれたが、最初の「代言人規則」は1876年に制定された。それによれば、代言人は、布告布達沿革の概略、刑律の概略、現今裁判手続の概略に通ずる者で、品行や履歴について地方官の検査をうけたうえで、司法卿の認可をうけるというもので、これが弁護士制度の開始である。

　これは1880年5月に改正されて、①代言人は検事の監督の下におく、②代言人組合を法定して、各地方裁判所本支庁ごとに一つの組合を設け、組合加入をすすめる。とされ、これが、現在の弁護士会

につながるのである。また、これによって代言人の試験についても、司法卿が所轄検事に問題（試験科目は、民事・刑事に関する法律、訴訟手続き、裁判の諸則）を送り、検事が担当することになった。

（2）弁護士法時代

1893年5月に弁護士法が施行された。司法省は、裁判所構成法とともに大審院・控訴院・地方裁判所ごとの所属弁護士とする三階級制や多額の免許料・保証金を内容とする制度を作ろうと目論んだが、不成功に終わった。しかし、弁護士会（地方裁判所ごとに一つ）を、検事正の強い監督下におくこと、司法大臣・裁判所より諮問された事項・司法若しくは弁護士の利害に関して司法省・裁判所に建議する事項以外議することはできないとすること、弁護士会には検事正を臨席させること、弁護士会の決議に司法大臣が無効だと宣言する権限・議事停止権を規定させたのである。

こうした官製の弁護士会に対して、鳩山和夫・磯辺四郎（東京弁護士会会長）・岸本辰雄（島根県、フランス留学、明治法律学校創設に参画）・菊池武夫（岩手県、アメリカ留学、わが国最初の法学博士）らが発起して、1896年日本弁護士協会を設立した。これは会員の親交、司法制度の発達、法律応用の適正を目的とするものであったが、結成されると、直ちに予審の廃止、あるいは予審に弁護人を付することを主張し、また起訴陪臣・検事制度などに付いて論じ合っている。

この弁護士の横の結合が、やがて官製の弁護士会をも巻き込みつつ、その後の重要な裁判闘争に意味をもち、日本の裁判闘争の質に影響を与えることになるのである。

ⅰ）足尾鉱毒事件

古河鉱業の銅山開発による排煙・毒ガス・鉱毒水によって周辺地域住民に重大な被害をもたらした足尾鉱毒事件において、1901年「生命救願請願人兇徒聚衆事件」がひきおこされ、52人が重罪・軽罪被告人にされた事件では、東京からの42人の弁護士に加え、横

浜・前橋・宇都宮からも16人の弁護士が加わり、総勢58人の弁護団を編成された。

ⅱ）日比谷焼打事件

　日露戦争後の講和に反対して起きた1905年9月5日のいわゆる日比谷焼打事件（兇徒聚衆罪）では、逮捕者2000余名のうち313名が起訴され、予審で有罪として公判に付されたもの117名におよんだ。194名が予審免訴となったが、2名が死亡した。このとき国民大会首謀者として、3人の弁護士が被告人になった。

　この事件で東京弁護士会は、警察官の良民殺傷の事実を重くみて会長ほか54人の弁護士を、東京全市を9地区に分けて調査し結果を公表したし、弁論では、任務分担して、総論主査には4人、結論主査に5人、個々人の被告に3人〜5人の弁護士をあて、群集心理で動いたとされる102名の弁護に100余名の弁護士がかかわった。こうして合計152名の大弁護団が編成されたのである。

ⅲ）大逆事件

　1910年の大逆事件、ほとんどデッチ上げの事件とはいえ、天皇への殺害計画とされる事件は、同年12月10〜29日大審院で傍聴禁止で16回の公判が行なわれ、翌年1月18日に公開で判決がだされた。この裁判でも、計11名の弁護士が被告の弁護を試みた。

　以上のような事件の弁護活動にとどまらず、明治末から大正初めにかけては、弁護士・弁護士会の監督を、検事正から司法大臣に移すことを求める運動、あるいは刑事法廷における弁護人の席を当事者対等の立場から検事席と同等にすることを求める運動をも弁護士協会は展開するが、これは実現に至っていない。ちなみに、検事が裁判官とならんで高壇に座るという形式は戦後の1947年まで続いた。

iv）米騒動

　さて、1918年の米騒動に際して日本弁護士協会は、8月19日、「今回ノ騒擾ハ政府ノ食料ノ問題ニ関スル施設徹底ヲ欠キ民心ノ帰響ヲ詳カニセザルニ因ル。吾人ハ速ヤカニ国民生活ノ安定ヲ図ルベキ根本政策ヲ確立スルノ要アリト認ム。騒擾ニ関スル司法権行使ハ其ノ措置ヲ誤ラザランコトヲ警告ス」と決議し、食料問題特別委員に16名、騒擾事件特別委員に16名、人権問題特別委員に16名、各特別委員会ごとに小委員5名ずつを選任するという布陣で臨み、静岡・愛知、山梨・長野・新潟、広島・岡山、京都・大阪・兵庫・三重、九州の5ブロックに分けて弁護士を派遣して調査、膨大な調査報告書をつくり、騒擾に軍隊を派出したこと、新聞雑誌への記事の掲載、演説会を禁じたことなどを批判する5つの決議を上げた。

（3）自由法曹団の結成

　これまでの事件は、非組織的な大衆運動における弁護活動であったが、米騒動以降に組織的・階級的運動が前進し、それがまた弾圧をうけた。ここでも、弁護団の活動が重要な役割を演じたのである。そして、その弁護団もその階級的姿勢を鮮明にするのである。

　1921（大正10）年6月から8月にかけて、三菱造船所神戸工場と川崎造船所が同時に争議をおこし、両者は、8時間労働制・組合の団体交渉権・横断的組合加入などを求める運動を展開した。その7月29日に川崎造船所の労働者1万3000人が生田神社で集会しデモを敢行した。ここに抜刀警察官が突入し、1労働者が背中から切りつけられて死亡するという事件が起きた。神戸弁護士会はこの問題を取り上げ、1弁護士に一任したが、東京弁護士会は直ちに、神戸人権蹂躙調査団結成協議会を結成して、16人の委員を神戸に派遣して、神戸弁護士会とともに調査を行ない、具体的な人権侵害の事実を明らかにして、神戸・大阪・東京で報告集会をおこなった。これらの弁護士を中心に10月ごろに「自由法曹団」が結成されたのである。「神戸人権問題調査報告書」の冒頭には、「大れ権利確保は法律の使命なり、而して生命身体の自由は基本的の権利なり」とあり、

これが調査団の最大公約数であり、自由法曹団もこの精神で結集したものと思われるが、自由主義者・社会民主主義者がここに結集したのである。
　大正デモクラシーを経験する中で、無産運動・社会主義運動が、天皇制国家の専制主義や戦争政策に反対する勢力として形をあらわしはじめる。これに対する弾圧法規として政府は、1925年治安維持法を成立させた。この治安維持法を使っての最初の大掛かりな共産党弾圧が、1928年の3・15事件であり、翌年の4・16事件であった。
　これに対して、解放運動犠牲者救援会が弁護士を中心に、労農大衆と進歩的インテリゲンチュアを糾合して結成され、1930年5月には国際労働者救援会（1922年創立、モップル）の日本支部となった（通称「赤色救援会」）。
　さらに、1931（昭和6）年4月29日に、3・15や4・16事件の法廷闘争（1931年6月25日に第1回公判）のために、解放運動犠牲者救援弁護士団が結成された。彼等は被告の弁護のための法廷闘争をおこなうとともに、岩田義道労農葬を主催したり、獄死させられた小林多喜二の死体引き取りなどをおこなった、
　その後、1931年に全農全国会議弁護団が結成されると、1933年には解放運動犠牲者救援弁護士団と全農全国会議弁護団が結合して、日本労農弁護士団結成される。かれらは、①資本家地主の階級裁判絶対反対、②治安維持法犯人の全部無罪、③在獄政治犯人の即時釈放、④白色テロル反対、⑤帝国主義戦争反対、⑥プロレタリア独裁社会主義ソヴェート日本樹立のために、をスローガンに掲げて、「社会運動通信」を発行し、東京のほか、横浜・水戸・前橋・静岡・新潟・名古屋・大阪・福岡・札幌・京城・台南に支部をつくった。
　しかし、その後日本労農弁護士団所属弁護士の一斉検挙が行なわれ、団の活動、弁護士としての活動そのものが、「治安維持法」第1条1項の「目的遂行罪」にあたるものとされた、かつ、予審終結決定では、解放運動犠牲者救援弁護士団・全農全国会議弁護団を日本共産党の拡大強化を目的とする「秘密結社」と認定して、その存在そのものを否定したのである。ここに自由法曹団・日本労農弁護士

団も壊滅するにいたる。

3）戦後日本社会と司法
（1）日本国憲法と戦後の裁判制度

　ポツダム宣言を受諾して無条件降伏した日本は、15年にわたる戦争でアジアの諸国と国民に甚大の犠牲を強い（2,000万人を殺害）、自らの国民にも大きな犠牲をもたらした戦争を、深く反省し、二度と戦争をしないことを決意し、平和的に生きる権利・基本的人権は人類普遍の権利であること、これを実現するためには主権が国民に存することを明確にして、日本国憲法を制定した。日本国民と日本国は、これを世界に宣言して、その実行を約束したのである。私たちの、人権と民主主義、そして平和追求の運動は、すべてここに由来する。

　日本国憲法は、三権分立主義を採用して、立法権を国会に（41条）、行政権を内閣に（65条）に属さるとともに、「すべて司法権は、最高裁判所及び法律の定めるところにより設置する下級裁判所に属する」（76条1項）と規定した。そして「すべて裁判官は、その良心に従ひ独立してその職務を行ひ、この憲法及び法律にのみ拘束される」と規定して、裁判官の独立、ひいては司法権の独立を宣言している。

　最高裁判所の下にある下級裁判所は、高等裁判所（8か所）、地方裁判所（都道府県に1か所づつ）、家庭裁判所（地方裁判所と同一の地に）及び簡易裁判所（警察署の1～2つを単位に、575庁）である。これらのうち、第1審裁判所は、原則として地方裁判所・家庭裁判所・簡易裁判所、第2審裁判所は、原則として高等裁判所で、第3審裁判所は、これも原則として最高裁判所である。何れも原則としての話で、例えば簡易裁判所の民事事件で地方裁判所が第2審として裁判をした事件については、高等裁判所が第3審裁判所となり、特別上告の申し立てが行なわれれば、最高裁は第4審となるのである。

（２）戦後復興と公害問題の発生

　日本の戦後は、荒廃の中から始まった。GHQ による占領政策の中で、政府は経済復興計画を担当する国家機関として 1946 年 8 月に経済安定本部を設け、12 月に「傾斜生産方式」を決定した。これは、壊滅的な日本経済を復興させるために、石炭や鉄鋼などといった基幹部門に資金や資材を集中し、全生産を軌道に乗せようというものであった。日本興業銀行の復興融資部を母体につくられた復興金融公庫（復金）は、石炭・鉄鋼・電力・肥料・海運などに集中的に融資をしたが、水俣の日本窒素はその対象となった。日窒の創業は 1908 年だが、政府の戦争政策の支援をうけて発展、しかし空襲をうけて破壊されていた。戦後の食糧増産と合わせての肥料増産の必要から、戦後政府からまたしても支援をうけて再興するのである。国家との結合をもって産業活動の使命と認識する企業は、その企業活動が環境を破壊し、地域住民・周辺住民の健康や生命に重大な影響を与えるであろうことに一顧だにしない、こうした形で経済復興が促進されたのである。

　この復興期につづく、高度経済成長期もまた、環境や健康はおおむね無視された。公害問題はこのようにして発生し深刻になった。企業は、生産力の拡大にのみ関心をもち、安全や環境保全のための投資をほとんど行ってこなかったこと、資源浪費型の重化学工業中心の産業構造の構築が行なわれたことなどによって、企業集積地域を中心に大気汚染、排水による水質汚濁が急速に進んだのである。日窒の工場廃水は何の処理もされないまま水俣湾に垂れ流され、有機水銀に侵された魚類を日常的に食する住民の命と健康を奪っていった。

（３）原因企業と地域住民と司法

　公害の深刻化に対して、政府は対症療法的には、1958 年に水質二法を制定し、1962 年には煤煙規制法を制定した。しかし、産業優先の姿勢を抑止するものとはならず、校外の深刻さに苦しむ被害者や地域住民を中心とした公害反対運動が、各地で展開され、地方自治

体を動かし、裁判所を動かし、国を動かすようになるのである。

　日本で初めて公害裁判に立ちあがったのは、第二水俣病といわれ、熊本の水俣病と同じ原因物質有機水銀によって被害をうけた新潟の人たちであった。原因企業は昭和電工鹿瀬工場で、阿賀野川に工場廃水を垂れ流して有機水銀中毒を引き起こしたのである。被害住民は1967年9月に新潟地方裁判所に提訴したのであるが、このたたかいが、四日市の石油コンビナートによる大気汚染、これによって呼吸系疾患に罹患した被害者らが同年9月に津地裁四日市支部に提訴につながり、1968年3月の、富山県のカドミウム中毒事件（原因企業は富山県神通川上流の二井金属神岡鉱山）での提訴（富山地裁）に、そして翌1969年6月の水俣病での提訴（熊本地裁）に発展するのである。

　これがいわゆる四大公害訴訟と呼ばれるものであるが、被害の程度やその規模（広範囲であること）などにおいて遥かに残酷で深刻であるにもかかわらず、裁判闘争に至るのに時間を要し、なおたたかい続けなけらばならないところに、原因企業と地域との関係、国家・地方行政との関係において、水俣病問題は深刻な解決されるべき問題を抱えていたといわなければならない。

　日窒は、水俣地域と住民の中に深く入り込み経済生活・社会生活など不即不離の関係が形作られ、そして水俣市行政とも分ちがたく結び付いていた（水俣は日窒の城下町とよばれた）。これはまた、地域の差別的構造とも連動していた。したがって、被害者が声をあげて企業を批判することはきわめて困難であった。

　したがって、裁判闘争は、様々なしがらみから自由になるためのたたかいでなくてはならなかったし、強い覚悟を要求された。

　しかし、水俣病の司法を舞台とするたたかいが、正義のたたかいとして、人間の尊厳と人権を勝ち取るたたかいとして、被害者と周辺のさまざまな人たちの共同のたたかいとして、さらに広範な知識人や心あり人たちを巻き込んで展開されたこと、そして一つひとつ成果を勝ち取ってきたことが、被害者自身の主体性を創り上げた大きな要因なのだが、ここでこのこれらの被害者と周辺を結合させる

要となり続けたのが、弁護士集団であった。1949 年公布の改正「弁護士法」によって「基本的人権を擁護し、社会正義を実現する」（第 1 条）ことを使命とする戦後の弁護士も、文字どおりこの精神を貫くことは容易ではないが、戦前からのたたかいの歴史の中で、弁護士集団はこの水俣病問題にかかわりつつ、それを実践してきたのである。

　水俣病問題を中心としたたたかいの歴史は、戦後日本の、人間の尊厳と人権、そして環境権と総称される、人間と自然が幸せに共生できる環境づくりにとって、重要な役割を演じ続けているのである。

1
水俣病の歴史

1）水俣病の発生

（1）水俣病発生の歴史

　水俣病は、日本列島の南側にある九州の熊本県水俣市で発生した水汚染公害です。発生した水俣市の地名から水俣病と言われています。原因物質は有機水銀の一種であるメチル水銀です。メチル水銀は、日本窒素株式会社（チッソと省略）という企業の水俣工場から排出された廃水に含まれていました。このメチル水銀が食物連鎖の中で魚介類に摂取されました。そして、メチル水銀によって汚染された魚介類を多食することによって、水俣病になります。

　1956年5月1日水俣病は公式に確認され、1965年には本州の半ば付近にある新潟（にいがた）県でも第2の水俣病(新潟水俣病と呼ばれる)の発生が公表されました。新潟での原因企業は昭和電工鹿瀬（かのせ）工場で、阿賀野川の上流に位置しています。

　公害対策の古典的な方法は、工場から排出される廃水を希釈（きしゃく、薄める）することです。しかし、水俣では、当初工場廃水が排出されたのは水俣湾です。しかも、この水俣湾は不知火海（しらぬいかい）という内海にある閉鎖水系です。新潟では、阿賀野（あがの）川という閉鎖水系でした。双方とも、メチル水銀が希釈しにくい閉鎖水系に工場が立地されていたのです。

　熊本県南端の小さな漁村であった水俣にチッソが進出したのは、1908（明治41）年でした。チッソは、その2年前に近くの鹿児島県大口に発電所を造りました。そこから生み出される豊富な電力と、

不知火海一円から採掘される石灰岩を原料にカーバイド製造等の電気化学工業を興し、さらにアンモニア、アセトアルデヒド、合成酢酸、塩化ビニール等の開発を進め、一大電気化学工業としてわが国有数の規模を誇る企業に発展しました。

チッソは第二次大戦の敗戦によって、朝鮮半島や中国等アジア各地の海外資本のすべてを失い、水俣の工場も、米軍の爆撃によって大きな損失を被りました。しかし戦後、政府からの復興支援によって、チッソは急速に発展し、水俣はチッソの企業城下町となっていきました。

水俣病の直接の原因となった水銀を触媒とするアセトアルデヒドの生産高は、1960（昭和35）年には45,000トンにも達しました。これは、全国シェアの25%から35%を占めるもので、チッソはわが国のトップ企業となっていきました。

アセトアルデヒドの大量生産を開始した1950年頃、水俣湾周辺ではさまざまな環境の変化が始まりました。水俣湾内の排水口に近いところから汚物が浮かび上がり、貝がいなくなりました。しばらくすると汚染は湾全体に広がります。湾の周辺では魚が大量に浮き上がり、またはふらふらと泳ぎ、貝は口を開けて死んでいました。陸上では猫が狂い回り、海に飛び込んでは死に、海鳥やカラスも飛べなくなり、地上をばたばた這って死んでいきました。住民は海水に異変が起こっているのではないかと不吉な予感に襲われながら、それでも暮らしていくために、海で魚をとっては食べ、売りに行く生活を続けました。

1956年4月21日、水俣沿岸で漁もする船大工の5歳の娘が、当時水俣地域では最も医療水準の高いとされていたチッソの附属病院に入院しました。女児は箸が使えず、歩くのもふらふらし、話し言葉もはっきりしない状態でした。そして、そのような症状の子どもが近所に何人もいるというのです。それを確かめたチッソ附属病院の院長細川一は、同年5月1日、「脳症状を主訴とする原因不明の患者が発生、4人が入院した」と水俣保健所に報告しました。なお、後にこの日が水俣病の公式確認の日といわれるようになりました。

この報告を受けて地元医師会などの関係機関による対策会議が開かれ、地域の医療機関のカルテを洗い出した結果、1953年12月に、やはり5歳の女児が発病していたことがわかりました。この患者が発生第1号とされています。しかし水銀を触媒とするアセトアルデヒドの生産は、1932年から始まっていました。だから実際には何の病気か分からないまま見過ごされていただけで、もっと前から発生していたという指摘もあります。

（２）患者発生の原因究明

　深刻な「奇病」発生ということで、熊本大学は医学部を中心に研究班を立ち上げました。熊大研究班では、患者を学用患者として入院させ疫学調査と病理解剖を行いました。その結果、1956年11月には「原因はある種の重金属」であり、人体への進入経路は「魚介類」であることを突きとめました。この時点で、人体に有害な物質が魚介類を通じて疾病を引き起こしているとして、魚介類の摂食禁止措置などの適切な措置がとられていたら、たとえ原因物質の特定や発症のメカニズムが解明できていなくても、患者の拡大は抑えられたでしょう。これが国や県の最初の、そして最大の失策です。

　汚染源はチッソ水俣工場が疑われましたが、チッソは有機水銀を含む無処理の排水を流し続けました。

　1959年7月、熊大研究班はついに有機水銀が原因と発表しました。チッソは直ちに、熊大研究班の有機水銀説は「科学常識から見ておかしい」と反論しました。その他にも、チッソも加盟する日本化学工業会は「戦後の爆薬投棄が原因」と発表、政府の意を受けた学者も「アミン中毒説」を発表するなど、さまざまな反論・妨害が行われました。

　その中で熊大研究班を中心とする厚生省食品衛生調査会水俣食中毒部会は、1959年11月、「水俣病の主因は水俣湾周辺の魚介類に含まれるある種の有機水銀化合物」との答申を厚生大臣に出しました。ところが厚生省は答申の翌日、この答申を認めたくないために逆に同部会を解散させました。その裏でチッソは熊大研究班に反論しな

がら、実は自らも工場排水を餌に混ぜてネコに与える「ネコ実験」をしていました。そしてそのネコ（400号と呼ばれます）が1959年10月に水俣病を発症しましたが、工場はこの事実を極秘にしたまま「原因不明」としていたのです。このように、熊大研究班などの原因究明に対して、チッソ、日本化学工業会、厚生省などは事実の隠ぺい・反論・妨害を行いました。

　しかし熊大研究班は研究を継続させました。翌年には熊大研究班は水俣湾産の貝から有機水銀化合物の結晶を抽出しました。さらに1962年8月にはチッソのアセトアルデヒド工場の水銀滓から塩化メチル水銀を抽出するなど、逃れようのない科学のメスが迫っていきました。熊大研究班は、1963年2月、「水俣病は水俣湾産の魚介類を食べて起きた中毒性疾患であり、原因物質はメチル水銀化合物であり」「それは水俣湾産の貝及びチッソ水俣工場のスラッジから抽出された」と発表し、科学的には結論が出ました。真理を探究する大学研究者の健闘の成果です。

　一方、さかのぼって国の対応に目を向けると、水俣病発生の初期は国（厚生省）は原因解明に乗り出しましたが、原因の究明がチッソに向けられるようになると、逆に原因隠しに向かいました。

　1956年に重金属説が発表されると、熊本県は「食品衛生法を適用し、水俣湾産の魚介類の採取を禁止したい」と厚生省に照会しました。これに対し厚生省は、国と県で半分ずつ費用補償しなければならないため、「水俣湾産の魚介類すべてが有毒化しているという明らかな根拠はないので適用できない」と回答しました。また、1958年に制定された水質保全法や工場排水規制法も適用せず、チッソの無処理廃水を放置し続けました。厚生省と科学技術庁がすなわち国が水俣病を「チッソ水俣工場からの公害である」と認めたのは、日本中からアセトアルデヒド工場が無くなった後の1968年9月のことでした。

（3）被害者へのチッソの不誠実な対応
　工場の廃水を無処理のまま排出していたのですから、チッソによ

る海洋汚染は工場設立当初から始まっていました。次第に汚染は深刻になり、大正時代にはすでに水俣漁協との間で漁業被害に対する補償協定が結ばれていました。しかし患者の発生が表ざたになったのは、公式確認がなされた 1956 年です。

その後もアセトアルデヒドの増産は続き、それに比例して患者は増加していきました。

水俣漁協は補償や原因の究明を求めました。そこでチッソは 1958 年に汚染が深刻な水俣湾に注ぐ百間排水口から、水俣川河口にある八幡プールを経て水俣川に排出するように排水ルートの変更を行いました。この事態に驚いた国は、排水ルートを 1959 年 11 月、元の百間排水口に戻させました。すなわち、チッソは汚染源に対しての原因究明の手を何も打つことなくその後もアセトアルデヒドの増産を続けたため、不知火海全域に水俣病の発生地域が拡大していきました。

このような事態の中でチッソは 1959 年 12 月 30 日、熊本県知事などの斡旋で初めて患者団体との協定を結びました。しかし、賠償というものではなく、あくまでも原因不明ということを前提に工場が患者にお見舞いをするという形のものであり、「見舞金契約」と呼ばれました。もっともチッソは、このとき既に、前述の「ネコ実験」によって自らが患者を発生させた犯人であることを知っていたのです。その内容は、①死亡者 30 万円などという低額補償、②水俣病の原因がチッソであると判明しても新たな補償はしない、③チッソが原因でないと判明したらこの補償も打ち切る、という極めて不当なものでした。

しかし、病気で働くこともできず、治療費にもその日の生活にも事欠く患者達は、ついにこの契約を結びました。後にこの契約は熊本第一次訴訟判決において「患者らの無知と経済的困窮状況に乗じて極端に低額の見舞金を支払い、損害賠償請求権を放棄させたもの」として、公序良俗に反し無効であると判断されました。

1959 年 7 月、熊大研究班の有機水銀説の発表等で水俣漁民は工場の廃水浄化を強く要求していました。これに対し、チッソは同年 12

月浄化装置のサイクレーターをつくり、これにより廃水はきれいになり、水俣病は終わると宣伝しました。完成式の記者会見で工場長はサイクレーターを通した廃水と称してコップの水を飲んでみせました。ところが、その水は単なる水道水であり、サイクレーターには水銀除去の目的も性能もないことが後に判明しています。結局、水俣病の原因となった有機水銀は浄化されることなく 1966 年に完全循環式になるまで排出され続けました。1968 年 5 月にアセトアルデヒドの生産を停止し、その 4 ケ月後に政府は初めて水俣病はチッソが原因の公害病だと認めたのでした。

2）裁判の経緯

（1）熊本水俣病第一次から第三次訴訟まで

　チッソの企業城下町といわれた水俣地域では、原因がチッソ工場からの汚水であることが分かっていても、チッソを相手に責任追及することは簡単なことではありませんでした。しかし、不誠実な対応をとり続けるチッソの姿を前に、正当な被害回復を求めるには裁判しかないと、患者らは裁判に訴えることにしました。

　熊本水俣病第一次訴訟（1969 年 6 月提訴）の大きな争点は、チッソの過失責任が認められるかどうかでしたが、熊本地裁判決（1973 年 3 月 20 日）は、チッソを断罪してその過失責任を認め、前述の「見舞金契約」についても公序良俗に反して無効であると判断し、患者 1 人当たり 1,600 万円〜1,800 万円の損害賠償を認めました。この画期的な判決後、チッソは患者団体との間で補償協定を結び、行政による水俣湾のヘドロ処理について仮処分が認められ、さらにチッソ社長らの刑事事件での有罪判決につながっていったのです。

　熊本水俣病第二次訴訟（1973 年 1 月提訴）の訴訟は、未認定患者の救済の皮切りとなりました。この時期、国は認定基準を厳しくし、かつ判断者は国が選んだ特定の医学者であるなど、「大量切り捨て政策」をとっていました。この国の認定基準は「昭和 52 年判断条件」と呼ばれ、複数の症状の組み合わせを水俣病認定の条件とし、感覚

障害だけでは認定しないという厳しい内容でありました。しかし、第二次訴訟に対しての 1979 年 3 月の熊本地裁判決は、この国の認定基準を採用せず、14 人中 12 人を水俣病と認めました。

さらに 1985 年 8 月の福岡高裁判決において、四肢の知覚障害だけでも汚染魚を多食しているなどの疫学条件が認められれば水俣病と認定しました。この判決は、「複数の症状の組み合わせを水俣病認定の条件とし、感覚障害だけでは認定しないという」国の厳しい認定基準と認定審査会を、「このような国の認定基準は破綻している」と批判したものでした。このような中で、国の「大量切り捨て政策」の問題点がクローズアップされました。

勝訴判決が続いても、国（環境庁）が認定基準を見直さない態度は変わりませんでした。原告や弁護団は、患者救済のためには国の責任を明らかにして国の政策を転換させる必要があると考え、熊本地裁への大量提訴（1,400 人）と全国的展開（新潟、東京、京都、福岡での提訴と全国連の結成）で、国と熊本県の責任を求める裁判すなわち熊本水俣病第三次訴訟(1980 年 5 月)を起こしました。1987 年 3 月、この熊本水俣病第三次訴訟第一陣に対する熊本地裁判決は、国と熊本県の責任を認めるという全面勝訴判決でした。その後、1990 年 9 月の東京地裁を皮切りに各裁判所で和解勧告がなされ、1993 年 1 月の福岡高裁和解案では、総合対策医療事業の治療費・療養手当プラス一時金（800 万円、600 万円、400 万円）という案が出されました。しかし、国は拒否しました。

その後、1993 年 3 月の熊本地裁第三次訴訟第二陣判決と同年 11 月の京都地裁判決においても国と熊本県の責任が認められ、「疫学条件があり、四肢末梢優位の感覚障害が認められ、他疾患によるものと明らかにできないものは水俣病である」と判断されたのです。このように各地裁や福岡高裁で国の厳しい認定基準は破綻しているという判決が何度も出されたにも関わらず、国は考えを変えていません。

そのような国の責任を認める地裁判決が相次ぎ、追い詰められた国（政府）は腰を上げ、1995 年 12 月に政府解決案を提案、翌年原

告団側はこれを受け入れ、チッソとも協定が結ばれました。この1996年政治解決とは、患者らをはっきり水俣病と認めず、国・熊本県の責任も曖昧なままの内容でしたが、原告の高齢化や大量原告の早期救済を図るため、後に結成されるノーモア・ミナマタ水俣病被害者・弁護団全国連絡会議（全国連）の原告らを含む11,000人の患者は政治解決を受け入れる選択をしたのです。

（2）関西訴訟最高裁判決（2004年10月）とそれ以降の動き

一方、かつて水俣湾周辺に居住し、その後関西方面に転居した水俣病患者によって結成された関西訴訟原告団は、政治解決ではなくあくまで裁判での判断を求めました。

2001年4月27日、関西訴訟控訴審判決（大阪高裁）は、チッソのみでなく国・熊本県の責任も認め、感覚障害だけで水俣病と認定しました。その後、2004年10月15日、最高裁判所は、大阪高裁判決を支持し、国・熊本県の責任を最高裁判所において確定したのです。最高裁は水俣病の病像について、この2001年大阪高裁の判断を是認しました。

その大阪高裁の判断とは、①水俣湾周辺地域において汚染された魚介類を多量に摂取したことの証明、②次の3要件のいずれかに該当するものであること、という基準でメチル水銀中毒を認定するという内容です。

　　（ⅰ）舌先の二点識別覚に異常のある者及び指先の二点識別覚に異常があって、頚椎狭窄などの影響がないと認められる者
　　（ⅱ）家族内に認定患者がいて、四肢末梢優位の感覚障害がある者
　　（ⅲ）死亡などの理由により二点識別覚の検査を受けていないときは、口周囲の感覚障害あるいは求心性視野狭窄があった者
すなわち最高裁も、感覚障害だけで水俣病と認めた大阪高裁の判断を承認したのです。

1996年政治解決によって、水俣病の問題は終わったとされていました。しかし、関西訴訟最高裁判決によって事態は一変しました。

なぜならば2004年関西訴訟最高裁判決が、国の厳しい判断基準よりも緩やかな条件で患者を水俣病と認定したため、これによって行政の認定基準が改められ、新たに救済を受けられるという期待が広がり、認定申請者が急増したのです。

しかし、国（環境省）は「最高裁判決は認定基準を直接否定してはいない」と逃げ口上で判断基準を改めようとしませんでした。結局、数次にわたる訴訟、そして最高裁判決を経ても、国は水俣病患者の根本的な救済を頑なに拒む態度を明らかにしたのです。このような国の態度を受け、国は裁判以外では動かないことを再認識した水俣病患者の人々の中から、国を直接相手取った裁判をすることによる救済を求めようとする人が増えていきました。

そして、2005年10月3日、新たに不知火患者会会員で結成された50名の原告団が、熊本地方裁判所に「ノーモア・ミナマタ国家賠償等訴訟」を新たに提起したのです。

2
「ノーモア・ミナマタ国家賠償等訴訟」
たたかいの記録

1）裁判で目指したもの

　ノーモア・ミナマタ国賠等訴訟は、司法制度を活用して、大量・迅速な被害者救済の実現を目指すものでした。前述の「1996年政治解決」により、約1万人の被害者が救済されました。しかし、それでもまだ多くの未救済被害者が存在していると考えられていました。というのも、濃厚汚染時に不知火海沿岸地域には約20万人の住民が居住しており、水俣湾周辺の汚染された魚介類を多食した被害者は多数存在していると思われるのに、全般的な汚染の実態調査が行われていなかったからです。また、「金ほしさのニセ患者」などという攻撃が加害者側から行われており、更には差別、偏見をおそれて名乗り出ない状況も続いていたのです。

　しかし2004年関西訴訟最高裁判決が言い渡され、その中で認定基準が改められたため、救済を受けられるのではないかとの期待が広がり、多くの人が認定申請に立ち上がりました。しかし、国はこの最高裁判決にもかかわらず、認定基準を改めず、十分な救済策も取りませんでした。本来、数万人に及ぶ被害者の迅速な救済は、立法や行政施策で対応すべきですが、そのような措置が取られなかったのです。

　水俣病不知火患者会が母体となり、2005年10月3日、国、熊本県、チッソを相手に、最初の50人が賠償を求める訴訟を熊本地方裁判所に起こしました。原告らは当初から、訴訟上の和解手続きによる大量・迅速な被害者救済の実現を目指しました。というのは、ほ

とんどの被害者は高齢であり、また未救済被害者は数万人いると考えられることから判決で解決することになると数十年かかることが予想され、それでは生きているうちには救えないような不合理な結果になってしまうからです。

　和解といえば足して二で割るようなイメージがありますが、水俣病の場合全く違います。水俣病の裁判史上、国が和解協議に応じたことは一度もありませんでした。水俣病第三次訴訟においても、当時の原告らが、「生きているうちに救済を」の合い言葉のもと、首相官邸前で何日も座り込むなどの必死の運動を展開しました。しかし、国は和解協議には一切応じなかったのです。国を和解のテーブルに着かせること自体がたいへん困難な課題でした。

　私たちは、かつて国が拒否の理由としていた行政の根幹論（国賠責任及び認定基準は行政の根幹にかかわる問題で、和解協議では解決できないとの見解）は、2004年最高裁判決により、根拠を失ったと考えました。そして、数万人に及ぶ被害者の迅速な救済を図る方法は、訴訟上の和解手続きしかないとの結論に達したのです。私たちの構想は、訴訟において医師団の診断書の正しさを徹底して証明し、大量提訴により解決を国に迫り、裁判所の和解勧告という決断を引き出し、協議を経て基本合意を行い、和解を実現するというものでした。

　第一陣提訴時、当時の環境大臣は、「和解はしない」と早々に拒否をしました。原告らはたいへん悲しい思いをしましたが、多くの支援と励ましを得て、5年半にわたるたたかいを続け、遂に2010年3月に基本合意、2011年3月に和解を実現したのです。

2）裁判闘争の記録

（1）原告団を拡大し団結を維持するたたかい

　私たち、ノーモア訴訟原告団の裁判は、2005年10月3日、前述した最初の50名すなわち第一陣原告団が熊本地方裁判所に提訴をするところから始まりました。その後、同年11月14日には第二陣

原告503名が提訴し、私たちの裁判は一挙にマンモス訴訟となりました。
　しかし、水俣病の場合、地域には複数の患者会が存在し、ノーモア・ミナマタ訴訟原告団の母体である水俣病不知火患者会は、人数においては最大の患者会ではありませんでした。そして、そのように複数ある患者会組織の中で、裁判によって正当な補償を求めようとする団体は、多数派ではありませんでした。
　私たちの裁判が始まると、当時の環境大臣は、「原告とは和解しない」と言い切り、裁判に対して強気の姿勢をにじませました。それは、裁判外での救済を求める団体の中には、政府が示す救済策を受け入れる姿勢を持った団体が複数存在し、かつそれらの団体に所属する被害者の方が数の上では優位に立っていたことからでした。
　私たちのたたかいはそのような政府の強硬姿勢を崩し、私たち裁判原告団を政府にとって「到底無視できない交渉相手」にするところから始まりました。

ⅰ）「すべての水俣病被害者の救済」を掲げての活動
　私たちは、不知火患者会会長であり、ノーモア・ミナマタ訴訟原告団長である大石会長がいつも口にする、「すべての水俣病被害者の救済」を旗頭に、私たちのたたかいこそがすべての被害者の救済につながるたたかいだと訴え、不知火患者会の会員とノーモア・ミナマタ訴訟の原告団を増やしていきました。
　いつの時代も、水俣病被害者にとって、情報は十分ではありませんでした。特に、現在の水俣病については、複数の補償制度が存在し、患者会の考え方も様々です。そんな中、自分にも水俣病の症状があるのではないかと考えた人たちが正確な情報を求め、多数不知火患者会に入会してきました。
　しかし、不知火患者会に入会する人たちすべてが、ノーモア・ミナマタ訴訟の原告になるわけではありませんでした。
　「裁判をする」ということは、被害者にとっては大変勇気のいることでした。私たちは、そのような抵抗感をなくし、多くの方に裁

判原告となってもらえるよう、2009年1月より、不知火患者会会員の戸別訪問を開始しました。私たちは、その活動を「ジョイント2009」と名付け、それまで約1,500名だった原告数を、約半年間で2,000名にすることを目指しました。同時に、近畿地方在住の被害者を中心に、大阪地裁への提訴も実現しました。原告数を増やすために、不知火患者会会員の戸別訪問、地域集会、裁判原告にも自分の親族や友人、知人で水俣病の症状がある人を裁判に誘うことを呼びかけました。また、地域に検診を呼びかけるビラの全戸配布、街頭での宣伝活動などをして、未だ声を上げられずにいる潜在被害者の発掘に努めました。

　また、これまでは取り組んでこなかった「対岸」の天草地域にも、未救済の被害者が多く残されているのではないかという予測のもと、同年4月1日には、上天草市龍ケ岳町樋島で住民対象の裁判説明会を実施しました。住民の大半が参加したのではないかと思われる100名を超える方々が参加し、裁判の説明に熱心に耳を傾けました。その後も各地で継続して集会を行いましたが、この樋島での集会は私たちに、天草地域での被害者の掘り起こしが必要だということを痛感させるものでした。これらの活動の結果、2009年7月末には、原告数を約1,900名にまで増やすことができました。

　原告数を飛躍的に増加させるきっかけとなったのが、2009年9月不知火海沿岸住民健康調査（大検診）でした。大検診は、水俣病患者7団体及び水俣病県民会議医師団、全日本民医連、地元医師会有志等で構成する実行委員会（実行委員長・原田正純熊本学園大学教授）が主体となって行われました。中でも不知火患者会は検診の呼びかけを大々的に行い、天草地域でも積極的に検診の受診者を募りました。

　大検診には、全国から約140名の医師が集まり、医療スタッフは実に約600名が参加しました。それらの医師やスタッフが、熊本、鹿児島両県の17会場に分かれ、2009年9月20、21両日で約1,000名の検診を行いました。大検診では、多数の潜在被害者が自らの症状を自覚し、補償を求めるに至ったという大きな収穫がありました

が、大検診がもたらしたものはそれだけではありませんでした。大検診に全国から多数の医師や医療スタッフが集まったことで、水俣病の診断についての理解が全国的に深まり、そのことが後の東京での提訴にもつながりました。また、不知火海沿岸地域から東京や大阪などの遠方に転居した被害者が、水俣病の検診や治療を受けることのできる医療機関も増え、被害者にとって大きな支えとなりました。

　私たちは大検診の後、裁判の説明会を各地で精力的に展開し、裁判こそが正当な補償を得るための唯一の方法であると訴えました。中でも、行政の線引きにより、保健手帳や水俣病認定申請者治療研究事業医療手帳（認定申請者に対して認定審査会の結論が出るまでの間の医療費の保障を行うため、原則として認定申請後1年経過後に発行される手帳）の交付を受けられない地域の被害者は、最後の望みを裁判に託す形で、提訴を決意していきました。その結果、大検診後の2009年11月18日に、私たちは原告数2,000名を突破することに成功しました。

　このようにして原告数を拡大しただけでなく、地域での説明会や集会を重ね、原告の団結を維持したことで、原告一人ひとりの中に裁判に対する確信が生まれてきました。

ⅱ）原告団の切り崩しとのたたかい

　2008年の年末から2009年にかけ、当時の水俣病問題与党プロジェクトチームは、救済水準としては極めて不十分な解決策を打ち出しました。さらには、2009年7月8日、チッソの分社化を主な内容とする水俣病被害者の救済及び水俣病問題の解決に関する特別措置法（特措法）が成立し、政府は私たち原告団の切り崩しにかかりました。

　しかし、原告団が、これによって切り崩されることはありませんでした。政府の思惑を、原告団の拡大を続けることと原告の団結を強めることで打ち破りました。そして、行政による線引きをものともせずに原告団を拡大し続けたことと、いかなる切り崩しにも屈す

ることなく原告団の団結を維持し続けたことは、政府にとっても脅威となり、原告団はもはや「無視できない集団」になったのです。

　特に、これまで水俣病の被害者は存在しないとされてきた天草の地域で多数の被害者が裁判に立ち上がったことは、政府にとっては脅威であったに違いありません。被害の拡がりが予測できないからです。もはや、原告団の勢いを止めるためには、原告団と交渉し早期に裁判を終結するしかありませんでした。

　このようにして「拡大」と「団結」に取り組んできたことで、「原告とは和解しない」と言い切った国の態度を変えさせることに成功しました。その結果、裁判は和解協議に入り、特措法に基づく救済水準も事実上、裁判で合意される形になりました。

　その後、東京地裁への提訴も実現し、たたかいは全国区のたたかいとなりました。原告団は名実ともに、水俣病被害者をリードする団体となったのです。

（2）争点と訴訟活動

ⅰ）争点としての病像

　ノーモア・ミナマタ訴訟では「原告一人ひとりが水俣病かどうか」が主な争点となりました。この争点は、具体的には次の3つに分けることができます。

　　①水俣病は、実態としてどのような病気であるのか（水俣病の症候）
　　②その実態を踏まえて、水俣病であるかどうかをどのようにして診断するのか（診察方法や診断基準など）
　　③その診断基準に照らして、原告一人ひとりは水俣病と診断できるのか

　この①と②はすべての原告に共通する問題（病像総論）であるのに対し、③は個別の原告についての問題（病像各論）であると言うことができます。

ⅱ）共通診断書の策定
　ノーモア・ミナマタ訴訟の原告の数は、2006年4月の時点で1,000名を超え、その後も増え続けることが予想されました。
　しかし、このような多数の原告について、一人ひとりが水俣病かどうかを裁判所に判断してもらうためには、気の遠くなるような長い時間がかかるのではないかとの心配がありました。そこで私たちは、診察の方法と診断書の書式を統一した「共通診断書」というものを用いることによって、迅速・適切な判断が可能であると主張しました。共通診断書とは、当時熊本学園大学で水俣学を担当されていた原田正純教授の呼びかけによって、長年にわたり水俣病患者の治療・研究に携わってきた医師ら有志が集まり、検討を重ねてまとめた水俣病の診断書です。そこに集まったメンバーの思いは、水俣病の共通診断書を策定することによって、水俣病被害者の迅速かつ適切な救済を実現したいという一点でした。その検討の結果、①水俣病の診断基準、②診断に必要な共通の診察の手順、③診断書の書式が完成したのです。
　したがって共通診断書は、現在の水俣病の診断に関する集大成とも言うべきものです。
　この共通診断書の特徴として、次の3点が指摘できます。
　第1に、これは一般的なメチル水銀中毒症の診断基準を提示するものではなく、あくまでも、チッソの排水による巨大な環境汚染によって引き起こされた公害病としての水俣病の診断に関するものだということです
　第2に、共通診断書の作成手順で示された水俣病の診断基準は、水俣病の病像が争われた過去の裁判の判決をも踏まえて策定されているという点です。すなわち、この診断基準の正しさは司法の場で既に確認されたものであり、裁判所における適切な被害救済につながる基準を提示したものなのです。
　第3に、多数の原告を迅速かつ適切に救済するのに必要十分な診察項目を厳選したという点です。この共通診断書に記載されている項目をチェックすることにより、原告一人ひとりが水俣病であると

診断できるし、被害の程度も把握できるよう工夫されているのです。
　私たちは原告全員について、この共通診断書の書式に基づいて個別の診断書を作成し、裁判所に提出することを決めました。原告一人ひとりが水俣病であることの立証は、この診断書だけで十分であると考えたのです。

ⅲ）高岡滋医師の証人尋問
　以上のような病像論や共通診断書が信用できるものであることを明らかにするために、私たちは、高岡滋医師の証人尋問を実施しました。高岡医師は長年にわたり、水俣病患者の診療および研究を水俣の現地で行うとともに、共通診断書の策定でも中心となられた方です。この重要な証人尋問は、2007年7月25日から始まり、主尋問3回、反対尋問四回を経て、2009年7月3日に終わりました。この2年間にも及ぶ証人尋問において明らかにされた水俣病の最新の病像論は、まさに水俣病の裁判史上に記録されるべき貴重な尋問となりました。
　そもそも水俣病は、人類が初めて経験した未曾有の公害病です。その実態については、不知火海沿岸地域で健康障害を訴える多数の患者の中から見出すほかありません。ところが、水俣病の全ぼうを明らかにする調査研究はきわめて不十分でしたが、藤野糺医師の桂島の疫学研究である「慢性水俣病の臨床疫学的研究」に代表される県民会議医師団等によって、水俣病の実態が明らかにされてきつつありました。
　高岡医師の証言では、こうした歴史や自身による最新の医学的研究結果をも踏まえて、水俣病においては四肢末梢優位の表在感覚障害や全身性の表在感覚障害などが極めて特徴的に認められ、メチル水銀曝露歴のある者にこれらの症候が認められれば、水俣病と診断できることが明らかにされました。これに対して国・熊本県、チッソは、「全身性の感覚障害というのは、大脳等の病理所見と矛盾するのではないか」などと主張しましたが、高岡医師は、病理所見にも限界があること、自分たちの観察や他の医師の観察でも全身性感覚

障害という現象が確認されており、その現象を非常に重視しなければならないことなどを反論しました。

　私たちが裁判所に提出した共通診断書は、診察の方法、正常・異常の判定方法、診断基準および診断書の書式が統一され、それに基づいて作成されています。

　高岡医師の証言では、感覚障害の診察には原則として筆と針による一般的な手法を用いること、感覚検査の数値化（定量化）や非汚染地域の調査等の研究成果を踏まえて診察方法と異常の判定を統一化したことで、所見の信用性が高められていることが明らかにされました。

　これに対して被告である国側は、「感覚障害の所見には客観性が乏しい」などと主張しましたが、高岡医師は、筆と針による感覚障害の有無のチェックは神経内科の基本であって、被告らの主張はまさしく医学の否定であると厳しく反論しました。

　また被告らは、高岡医師の考え方について「医学的にコンセンサスを得ているか」とか「教科書に載っているか」などと繰り返し質問しましたが、高岡医師は、水俣病の臨床疫学的な研究はほとんどなされておらず教科書といえるものはないこと、多くの医師にとって国の定めた「昭和52年判断条件」すなわち国の厳しい認定基準の存在が、広汎な被害実態を明らかにするための臨床研究の妨げになっていることなどを反論しました。

　水俣病の被害を矮小化する昭和52年判断条件に固執するあまり、現実をみようとしない被告らの不合理な態度が、まさに浮き彫りになった証言でありました。

　高岡医師は、第一陣原告50名について、共通診断書やその元となる問診票、カルテなどを踏まえて、全員を「水俣病である」と証言しました。

　これに対して被告らは、原告らの病気は「他の疾患や要因によるものである」などと主張しましたが、高岡医師は、共通診断書の書式自体が他疾患との鑑別ができるだけの項目を備えているだけでなく、共通診断書作成にあたって医師が十分な鑑別診断を行っている

ことを明らかにするとともに、ずさんな鑑別診断の主張をしているのはむしろ被告らの方であると反論しました。

　以上のような高岡医師の証人尋問を通して、共通診断書の信用性が裏付けられたことは、その後の被告らとの和解協議におけるルール作りにおいて大きな力を発揮しました。被告らは、和解のルールとして「救済対象者の判定資料は、共通診断書ではなく、被告側が指定する医師の診断による公的診断書を基礎とすること」を考えていたようですが、最終的には「共通診断書と公的診断書の双方を対等の判断資料とすること」に合意しました。これは、共通診断書に記載された医師の所見が信用できることを前提としたルールであり、高岡医師の証人尋問が成功していなければ実現できなかったものです。

　このように、高岡医師尋問は、水俣病被害者の救済を実現するにあたって大きな成果を上げました。

ⅳ）藤木素士博士の破綻（2009年11月13日証人尋問）

　ノーモア・ミナマタ訴訟では、水俣病の病像という争点のほかに、消滅時効や除斥期間（民法第724条）の規定により、国・熊本県・チッソが損害賠償責任を免れるかどうかも重要な争点となりました。

　国・熊本県は、裁判が始まってから約1年後の2006年11月20日の段階で、原告に水俣病の症状が発症してから20年を経過したことになり除斥期間が経過するため、国・熊本県は損害賠償責任を負わないと主張しました。また、チッソにおいても、2006年9月28日の段階で、国・熊本県と同様に20年の除斥期間を主張し、さらに水俣病第一次訴訟以来一度も主張しなかった「3年の消滅時効の経過」を突如持ちだし、これを理由に損害賠償責任を負わないと主張しました。

　特にチッソは、原告らに対して「関西訴訟最高裁の結論を見て気が変わったとしか言いようのない原告らの突然の請求は（中略）到底許されるものではない。1996年全面解決（1996年政治解決のことを意味していると考えられる）に至るまで長い間被告チッソに対し

賠償や補償を求めてきた人々と、いわば権利の上に眠るがごとく日を過ごし全面解決の時ですら何ら行動を起こさずに今になって突然訴訟を提起する本件原告らとを時効・除斥の観点で、同列に論じることこそ、著しく合理性を欠いている」と述べ（2007 年 4 月 27 日付け準備書面（4））、消滅時効と除斥期間を全面的に主張しました。これらの主張は、原告らが水俣病患者あるいは水俣病被害者であったとしても、時の経過のみを理由にして、国・熊本県・チッソが、責任から逃れようとするもので許し難いものでした。

　このような国・熊本県・チッソの主張は、2004 年関西訴訟最高裁判決でも一定の範囲で認められた除斥期間についての判断を、根拠とするものでした。すなわち、この判決は、水俣地方から関西地方などの遠方に転居した原告らについて、「転居の時から 24 年以内に認定申請をしなかった場合」には、仮に、その原告が水俣病被害者であったとしても、除斥期間により国・熊本県は損害賠償責任を負わないとの判断を示したのです。

　この判決における判断は、差別や偏見に苦しみ、症状があっても水俣病被害者として名乗りを上げることができない被害者の現実を見ないものであり、極めて不当というほかありません。だが、現実にはこの判決でこの点が判示されており、さらに裁判では多くの裁判官が最高裁判所の前例に従う傾向が強いことから、ノーモア・ミナマタ訴訟でも、除斥期間の問題が重要な法律上の争点となることが予想されました。

　国・熊本県は、高岡滋医師の証人尋問への反撃のために、藤木素士証人の尋問を用意しました。この藤木証人は、もともと微量の水銀の測量に関する研究者でした。ノーモア・ミナマタ訴訟において、水俣湾の魚介類に含まれる水銀濃度、住民の毛髪に含まれる水銀値、住民の新生児の臍帯（へその結）に含まれる水銀値などの調査結果に基づき、「アセトアルデヒドの生産を停止した 1969 年年以降は水俣病を発症するだけのメチル水銀による汚染はない」との証言をしました。実は藤木証人は、いわゆる水俣病第三次訴訟の時から国側の証人として、「1955 年頃における科学的知見からすれば、国や熊

本県が水俣病の被害拡大についての責任を負う必要がない」、つまり、国・熊本県の責任論を否定する根拠を証言し続けてきた人物でもありました。

　彼のノーモア・ミナマタ訴訟においての1969年以降水俣病は発症し得ない程度の汚染しかなかったことの主張を通して、原告の全員につき20年間の除斥期間が経過した根拠となる証言を行いました。

　藤木証人の「1969年以降には水俣病を発症しうるほどの汚染はない」との証言も、実際に1969年以降に生まれた住民にも水俣病症状がみられるという医師らの見解を真正面から封じることはできませんでした。

　ノーモア・ミナマタ訴訟は勝利和解により終結したため、藤木証人の見解についての裁判所の判断は示されませんでしたが、2011年の和解解決において、時の経過を理由に和解拒否された原告はいないこと、また、1969年以降に生まれた原告も、一部ではありますが水俣病被害者として和解の対象となったことからして、藤木証人の証言は全面的に否定されました。

　ノーモア・ミナマタ弁護団では、消滅時効、除斥期間の争点につき、他の訴訟の事例をもとにシンポジウムも開きました。また、複数の学者・弁護士の援助を得て、水俣病の原因究明を妨害し被害を隠し込んできた加害者側の態度からすれば、時効・除斥の主張自体が権利の濫用であること、さらに、時効や除斥の起算点を診断時や認定時と捉えて、すべての水俣病被害者に対する賠償を認めるべきであるとの準備書面を提出しました。

　しかし、時効・除斥の争点を突破するための最も本質的なポイントは、「未だに救済されていない水俣病被害者が多数存在することを社会的に明らかにすること」にほかなりませんでした。その意味で、最終的に3,000名規模に原告団を組織した原告団の拡大、及び、確固たる団結維持の取り組みと、医師団・支援の結束による水俣病患者掘り起こし運動、とりわけ、2009年9月20、21日にわたり、合計1,044名を対象に行われた不知火海沿岸住民健康調査（前述の大検診）の成功こそが、国・熊本県・チッソらによる時効・除斥の主

張を突破する最大の鍵となりました。

3）全国的な運動の展開

（1）水俣病は終わっていない〜全国縦断ミナマタキャラバン〜

　いうまでもなく私たちのたたかいは、2004年関西訴訟最高裁判決を契機に立ち上がった被害者らが起こしたものでした。しかし、1996年政治解決で多数の水俣病被害者らの救済が図られたことから、全国的には、水俣病は終わったとの認識が一般的でした。私たちのたたかいは、その世論を動かし、今なお水俣病の被害者が多数取り残されており、その救済を図る必要があるということを周知するところから始まりました。そこで私たちは、2008年5月16日から約2ヶ月をかけて、熊本から北海道まで、「水俣病は終わっていない」を合い言葉に、全国縦断ミナマタキャラバンを実施しました。

　キャラバンの出発式の日は、ノーモア・ミナマタ訴訟の第13回口頭弁論で、原告団の大多数を診断した高岡滋医師の証人尋問が採用され、裁判が大きな一歩を踏み出した日でもありました。キャラバンには、原告団、弁護団だけでなく、水俣病闘争支援熊本県連絡会議に所属する看護師も参加し、熊本地裁前から出発した全国キャラバン参加原告の体調の悪化にも備えました。

　2008年5月18日の福岡県を皮切りに、第1弾は広島県、岡山県、兵庫県、大阪府、京都府、愛知県、神奈川県の8府県をまわり、県庁訪問や支援団体への支援のお願い、街宣活動などを精力的に行いました。参加した原告は、「感覚障害」という見た目では分からない水俣病の症状を具体的に訴えました。被害者の生の声は、水俣病を知らない人々に衝撃を与え、公式確認から50年経ってもなお、水俣病被害者が、苦しみの中にいることを印象づけました。各地のマスコミも、キャラバンを取り上げて報道しました。その関心の高さには、私たち自身が驚かされるほどでした。そして、2008年6月2、3日の全国公害被害者総行動を中間地点とし、6月12日からキャラバンの後半戦がスタートしました。後半は、東京での念入りな訴えの

後、千葉県、埼玉県、茨城県、栃木県、群馬県、新潟県、福島県、山形県、岩手県、青森県の10県を経て、北海道入りしました。
　私たちが北海道を目指したのは、2008年7月に北海道において洞爺湖サミットが開催されることから、サミットの議長国である日本で、50年以上にわたり解決されない公害問題があるということを世界に発信するためでした。もちろん、サミット会場に入ることはできませんが、北海道までキャラバンをつなぎ、札幌での国際シンポジウムや、大通公園でのリレートークに参加しました。熊本からは遠く離れた北海道の地で、「水俣病は終わっていない」ことをアピールし、約1ケ月半に及んだキャラバンは成功裏に幕を閉じました。キャラバンも後半になればなるほど周知されるようになり、マスコミにも大きく取り上げてもらえるようになりました。そして、キャラバンで得たものは、全国的な支援の獲得だけではありませんでした。参加したすべての原告が、これまで人には話せなかった水俣病の被害を語ることが人々の共感を呼び、大きな支援につながることを実感し、自信を付けたことも大きな収穫でした。全国の仲間とともにこのようにして、運動体としての力を付けた私たちは、その後も現地での宣伝行動や原告団拡大の運動など、積極的な活動を続けることになりました。
　全国的な活動としては、全国の公害、薬害などの被害者団体が集い、関係省庁や加害企業との交渉や決起集会、街頭でのデモ、宣伝活動などを行う、全国公害被害者総行動（総行動）にも毎年参加しました。そして、水俣病問題は、総行動においても中心的な課題として取り上げられるようになりました。総行動への参加は、私たちと同様に公害や薬害の被害に苦しむ被害者らとの連帯を強固なものにし、全国的な運動の大きな足がかりとなるものでした。

（2）特措法による幕引きを許さない
　2009年7月8日には、「水俣病被害者の救済及び水俣病問題の解決に関する特別措置法（特措法）」が成立しましたが、この特措法の成立を阻止するための活動も、私たちのたたかいを大きく前進させ

るものでした。

　特措法は、当時の水俣病問題与党プロジェクトチームが提案した救済策について、私たち不知火患者会が明確にこれを拒否したことで、肝心の一時金の支払者チッソが、「最終解決にならない」と言って拒否したため、あらたに考案された法案でした。法律の名称は、水俣病被害者の救済をうたっていますが、被害者救済の内容は極めて不十分であり、実質的には加害企業チッソの分社化のための法案でした。被害者救済の内容は極めて不十分というのは、水俣病の加害責任が確定した国が被害者を選別するという制度を認めれば、被害者の大量切り捨てにつながることは明らかでした。一部の被害者団体はこれを歓迎しましたが、私たちは、これを被害者救済とは名ばかりの加害者救済、被害者切捨法案だとして認めることはできませんでした。

　私たちは、特措法の法案が与党案として浮上してきた2009年3月から、これを阻止する行動を始めました。まず、チッソ分社化がいかに許されないことかを訴えるため、同年3月4日、熊本市内で緊急シンポジウムを開催し、東京経済大学の除木理史准教授が分社化のスキーム（枠組み、ねらい、意味）について分かりやすく講演しました。

　また、原告団の団結をより強固なものにするために、ちょうど高岡医師の証人尋問が行われた同年3月13日には、尋問の昼休みの時間を利用して「特措法の国会上程に抗議する緊急集会」を開催し、特措法による解決には応じず、裁判を継続していくこと及び国会議員に私たちの考えを訴えていくことを確認しました。

　この頃から私たちは、度々上京し、国会議員に対し、水俣病問題の正当な解決を訴えていきました。6月2日には緊急の院内集会を行い、多数の野党議員が参加して私たちとの連帯を約束してくれました。しかし、当時野党であった民主党は、それまで熊本地方区選出の参議院議員が座長を務めていた「民主党水俣病対策作業チーム」の座長を解任し、民主党幹部に引き上げ自民党との合意を目指すようになりました。そのような民主党の動きにより、特措法の成立が

いよいよ現実的なものとなってしまいました。
　私たちは、最後まで諦めずに特措法の不当性を訴えるため、6月25日から国会前での座り込み行動を始めました。さらに環境委員会所属の国会議員を中心に要請行動を行い、合わせて、国会前での宣伝行動も継続していました。私たちの行動には、様々な方が賛同してくれました。中でも、環境大臣が2005年に設けた水俣病問題懇談会の委員であった柳田邦男氏や加藤タケ子氏が特措法に反対する意見を表明したことは、特措法の不合理性を社会にアピールすることになりました。
　特措法に反対する患者団体も連帯しました。このときの運動に共同して取り組んだ新潟水俣病阿賀野患者会とは、その後ノーモア・ミナマタ水俣病被害者・弁護団全国連絡会議（全国連）を結成し、和解まで共同してたたかうこととなりました。私たちへの支援の輪も、目に見える形で大きなうねりとなっていきました。座り込みを続けたことで、毎日、国会議員や支援団体の幹部、他の公害被害者など、多数の方々が応援に駆けつけてくれました。このときの連帯が、東京での支援の輪を広げ、後の東京提訴に大いに役立ったことは間違いありません。
　特措法は、私たちの徹底的な反対を押し切り、2009年7月2日には自民党、公明党、民主党の三党合意に至り、7月3日には衆議院で、7月8日には参議院でそれぞれ可決され、成立しました。私たちは、特措法の成立に憤りましたが、皮肉にも特措法が成立したことで水俣病問題が全国的に報道され、社会の関心を得ることになり、水俣病問題の解決が国政の重要課題となりました。また、特措法を阻止する運動と、民主党の水俣病対策作業チームに所属していた国会議員らの熱心な説得により、特措法の内容をより被害者救済に資するものとすることもできました。

（3）特措法成立後のたたかい

　特措法を巡るたたかいで、私たちは、最後まで諦めずにたたかうことが大きな成果を生むことを学びました。このとき、特措法は水

俣病被害者の救済の枠組みを定めただけで、救済内容はまだ白紙の状態でした。私たちは、裁判外の被害者のためにも、よりよい救済内容を勝ち取る必要がありました。私たちは、被害者救済の水準をよりよいものとするために、特措法成立後も継続して上京し、私たちの考えを伝える通信を作成して国会議員らに訴えました。原告団を拡大する運動も続け、首都東京での提訴も実現しました。

　それらの活動の一つの集大成が、2011年勝利和解であったことは間違いありません。

　しかし私たちのたたかいがこれで終わるわけではありません。「すべての水俣病被害者の救済」をかかげ、未救済の被害者がいる限り、私たちはたたかい続けるでしょう。そして、水俣病の教訓を国内だけでなく、世界に発信していかなければなりません。

3

2011年勝利和解の内容と成果

1) 和解所見による基本合意まで

　2009年7月8日に水俣病特別措置法が成立したことを受け、私たちは、「水俣病被害者をもれなく救済するのはやっぱり司法」であることを明らかにしながら、国・県・チッソに対し、裁判上の協議に基づく早期和解を求めていくことにしました。

　ノーモア・ミナマタ訴訟においても、被告らは、「感覚障害だけでなく複数の症状がなければ水俣病とは認めない」、「四肢末梢優位の感覚障害でなければ水俣病特有の症状とは言えない」など、水俣病像を狭く捉える考え方に固執していました。ところが、高岡滋医師の証人尋問をふまえ、特措法では、感覚障害だけでも水俣病とし、全身性の感覚障害も水俣病として認めざるを得なくなりました。

　また被告らは、「原告らは訴え出たのが遅すぎる」などとして、消滅時効・除斥期間による制限を主張していました。ところが、増え続ける被害者の前に、特措法では、期間による制限を設けることは出来ませんでした。

　こうして、被告らが訴訟で主張していた大きな2つの争点は、特措法の制定によって実質的に決着を見ました。そこで原告団は、同年7月31日に69名の追加提訴を行うとともに、同年8月9日には1,200名で決起集会を開き、「今こそ、被告らは、裁判上の協議に基づく早期和解のテーブルに着け！」とのたたかいを展開していくことを決議したのです。

　同年8月23日には水俣市で、熊本、近畿、新潟の原告団・弁護団

と東京の弁護団が、「ノーモア・ミナマタ被害者・弁護団全国連絡会議（以下「全国連」）」を結成しました（のちに東京原告団も加盟）。全国連は、全国の潜在患者を救済するうえで大きな役割を果たすとともに、その後の和解協議を共同歩調で進める際にも重要でした。

同年9月20、21日、不知火海沿岸17会場で、1,000人を対象とした沿岸住民健康調査が実施されました（原田正純実行委員長）。詳細は先に述べたとおりですが、この健康調査の結果は、それまで行政が「水俣病被害者はいない」としていた地域や世代にも多くの被害者が埋もれていることを社会的に明らかにし、被告らを震撼させました。

そして国は同年11月、ついに、裁判上の和解に向けた原告団との事前協議を開始せざるを得なくなりました。事前協議では主に、補償内容や判定方法について協議を重ね、論点を整理していきました。そして、2010年1月22日、熊本地方裁判所（高橋亮介裁判長）から当事者双方に対し、解決に向けた和解勧告が出され、ただちに和解協議に入りました。和解協議では、補償内容や判定方法のほか、対象地域や年代をどうするかについても、双方の考えを裁判所に訴えました。

一方、2009年2月27日に近畿在住の被害者12名が大阪地裁に提訴したのに続いて、熊本地裁で和解協議が開始された直後の2010年2月23日、関東在住の被害者23名が、東京地裁に提訴しました。近畿と東京での提訴は、和解協議のスピードを加速させるとともに、県外転居者救済の必要性を国につきつけることになりました。

3回の和解協議を経て、熊本地裁は2010年3月15日、解決所見を示しました。解決所見は、後で述べる和解の骨子となるものですが、三本柱（一時金・医療費・療養手当）の救済内容をはじめ、第三者委員会による判定方式、地域外原告を含む判定方法など、幅広い救済を求める原告らの意見を組み入れたものでした。原告団は、ただちに29地域で集会を開き、計1,000名を超える原告の参加で、解決所見について協議しました。そのうえで同年3月28日、水俣市総合体育館で1,050名の参加をもって総会を開き、圧倒的多数の賛

成で解決所見の受け入れを決めました。そして、被告らも解決所見の受け入れを決めていましたので、同年3月29日、熊本地裁で和解に向けた基本合意が成立したのです。

2）判定作業から和解成立まで

　原告団は、原告全員に第三者診断の意義やその後の手続を理解してもらいながら、第三者診断に臨みました。第三者診断前に死亡した原告でも、生前に公的検診を受けていればその結果を用いることで救済対象になりうることも交渉で勝ち取りました。

　御所浦を除く天草など、いわゆる対象地域外の原告については、水俣湾周辺の魚を多食したことについての資料作成・収集を行いました。

　弁護士が原告一人ひとりから話を聞き、供述録取書という形でまとめ上げたうえで、弁護士立ち会いのもと熊本県、鹿児島県の担当者が原告からヒアリングを行いました。

　第三者委員会は、座長の吉井正澄氏（元水俣市長）のほか、原告推薦の医師2名、被告推薦の医師2名の計5名で構成され、診断結果や疫学資料をもとに、毎回、熱心かつ公平な討議がなされました。第三者委員会の判定結果をふまえ、30地域で集会を開き、計1,700名を超える原告の参加で、和解の可否について協議しました。そして、2011年3月21日、芦北スカイドームで1,512名の参加をもって総会を開き、圧倒的多数で和解することを決めました。次いで、3月24日に東京地裁、25日に熊本地裁、28日に大阪地裁でそれぞれ和解が成立したのです。

3）和解の内容

　補償内容は、①医療費、②療養手当、③一時金の三本柱の給付です。

　①医療費については、健康保険の自己負担分を国・県が補助する

ことにより実質無料化され、一生涯、安心して医療を受けることができます。
　②療養手当は、入院した場合月額17,000円、通院の場合70歳以上なら15,900円、70歳未満なら12,900円です。これも生涯給付という点では、大変大きな補償です。
　そして、③一時金210万円に加え、団体一時金34億5,000万円（近畿・東京を含む）が支給されました。一時金の額は、2004年関西訴訟最高裁判決の水準に達しませんでしたが、医療費、療養手当を含む三本柱の給付となったこと、提訴から5年半という比較的短期間で勝ち取ったことを考えれば、原告団のたたかいの大きな成果と評価できます。
　環境省の環境保健部長は、「受診者がうそをついても見抜けない」「不知火海沿岸では、体調不良をすぐ水俣病に結びつける傾向がある」「カネというバイアスが入った中で調査しても、医学的に何が原因なのかわからない」など、あたかも原告らが「ニセ患者」であるかのごとき暴言で物議を醸しましたが、水俣病被害者と認めさせたうえでの和解を勝ち取ったことも、原告らにとっては大切なことです。
　基本合意で、「被告らが責任とおわびについて具体的な表明方法を検討する」とされていたことをふまえ、2010年5月1日、内閣総理大臣として初めて当時の鳩山由紀夫首相が水俣病犠牲者慰霊式に参加し、「水俣病の被害の拡大を防止できなかった責任を認め、改めて衷心よりお詫び申し上げます」と述べ、熊本県知事も同様に謝罪しました。
　なお、「国は、メチル水銀と健康影響との関係を客観的に明らかにすることを目的として、原告らを含む地域の関係者の協力や参加の下、最新の医学的知見を踏まえた調査研究を行うこととし、そのための手法開発を早急に開始するよう努める」と和解調書に明記させたことは、「すべての水俣病被害者の救済」を目指す不知火患者会にとって、不知火海沿岸住民の健康調査を実施させる足がかりとなるものです。

4）裁判上の和解の意義

　今回の和解は、給付内容もさることながら、大きく4つの点から評価できます。

　第1に、今回の和解は、40年に及ぶ水俣病裁判史上初めて、国を裁判上の和解のテーブルに着かせ、原告団と一緒に解決策を模索させた結果、勝ち取った点です。2004年関西訴訟最高裁判決で、水俣病の拡大に関する国と熊本県の法的責任が断罪されるとともに、国の厳しい認定基準が事実上否定されたことを受け、原告50名が、2005年、熊本地裁にノーモア・ミナマタ訴訟を提起し、「裁判所で協議して大量の被害者を早期に救済するためのルール（司法救済制度）を決めるべき」と提案しました。仮に、水俣病として補償を受けるべき被害者が50名しかいなかったとすれば、全員について判決を目指すとの方針をとることもあり得たかもしれません。しかし、2005年第一陣原告が提訴した時点で、すでに1,000名を超える被害者が熊本県と鹿児島県に対して認定申請をしており、まだまだ名乗り出ていない潜在患者が多数いることは明らかでした。そこで私たちは、数千、あるいは数万単位の被害者を早期に救済するためには、国、熊本県、チッソと、2004年関西訴訟最高裁判決に沿って和解することが必要かつ可能と考え、司法救済制度の確立を提案したのです。

　これに対し、2005年第一陣提訴当時の環境大臣は、「原告らとは和解しない」と言い放ちました。しかし国は、2009年、水俣病特別措置法の制定後も増え続ける原告団に対し、「原告とは裁判上の和解によって解決を図る」と方針転換せざるを得なくなり、特措法の具体化より先に原告団との和解のルールを決めるための協議を重ねたのでした。裁判上の和解を目指す以上、和解内容について原告団の納得が不可欠となり、ここに特措法による一方的な判定との大きな違いを生み出しました。その結果、第三者委員会による判定という、大量の原告を早期かつ公正に救済するためのルールを作り上げることができ、近畿・東京も含む2,992名の原告のうち2,772名（92.6%）

が一時金等の対象となり、医療費のみの対象者22名とあわせ93.3%の救済を勝ち取ることができたのです。

　第2に、行政単独の被害者選別を廃止させ、「第三者委員会」を加えた点で画期的です。

　これまで、「『誰が被害者か』については、行政（の指定した医師）が決める」というのが、国の一貫した政策でした（「行政の根幹」論）。これに対し、原告団は、「最高裁判決で加害者と断罪された国が、『誰が被害者か』を決めるのはおかしい」と批判しました。そして、高岡滋医師の証人尋問を実施し、県民会議医師団による「共通診断書」の信用性を明らかにしました。その結果、熊本地裁の解決所見は、委員の半数の人選を原告側に委ねる「第三者委員会」による判定方式を採用したうえ、県民会議医師団が作成した「共通診断書」を第三者（公的）診断結果書と対等に判定資料とすることとしました。すなわち、「誰が水俣病被害者か」についての判断権についての行政の独占を突破したのです。

　また、国(行政)がこだわってきた病像においても、全身性の感覚障害も水俣病と認めさせるなど、救済対象を広げました。これらは、他の公害被害者・薬害被害者認定の場面においても、大きなインパクトを与えるものといえるでしょう。

　第3に、天草をはじめ、これまで対象地域外とされてきた地域でも、約7割という高い救済率を勝ち取り、事実上、対象地域を大きく広げたものと評価できます。これまで行政は、行政区域で線を引き、地域外の者については、メチル水銀の曝露がないとして、救済を拒んできました。しかし、魚介類の摂取状況に関する供述録取書の作成や県のヒアリングへの立ち会い、ねばり強い和解協議を通じて、これまで行政が「水俣病の被害者はいない」としていた地域に多数の被害者がいることを認めさせたことは、地域外での特措法による救済の道を大きく開いたといえます。また、これまで1968年末までに出生した者に限っていた曝露時期についても、1969年11月30日生まれまでに拡張させるとともに、それ以降についても、一定の条件で対象者にすることができました。こうして、地域や年代に

よる線引きを突破したことは、「すべての被害者救済」に向けての大きな成果です。

　第4に、時効・除斥なき救済を勝ち取った点でも画期的です。チッソは原告らに対し、「権利の上に眠る者は保護に値しない」などとして時効による賠償請求権の消滅を主張し、国、熊本県も、すでに水俣病を発症して20年以上経つのだから、除斥期間によって権利主張が認められないなどと主張しました。じん肺（労災）や肝炎（薬害）などの裁判では、除斥期間によって原告の権利主張が制限されることがあります。しかし、ノーモア・ミナマタ訴訟においては、「公害に時効なし」との立場から、「原因企業であるチッソが消滅時効の主張をすること自体信義則に反し許されない」ことを裁判所の内外で明らかにするとともに、国・熊本県による除斥期間の主張についても、「水俣病の診断の難しさ、差別・偏見が根強いもとで水俣病として名乗り出ることの困難さを考えれば、発症してすぐに訴え出ることがいかに大変であるか」を明らかにしてたたかいました。そして、大量の被害者を前に、国は、水俣病特措法において除斥期間を設けることができず、ノーモア・ミナマタ訴訟においても除斥期間による差別をいうことはできなくなったのです。

　以上4点が、ノーモア・ミナマタ訴訟のたたかいの成果です。

むすび

水俣病問題の今後

　環境省は、2012年7月31日、水俣病被害者救済特別措置法（水俣病特措法）による水俣病救済策の申請を終了した。この段階までに申請者は65,151人に及んだ。しかしながら、行政は、申請者の処分の内容を明らかにしようとしない。しかし、チッソの2013年3月期連結決算などから、チッソが特措法の対象者のうち27,770人に一時金210万円を支払っていることが判明している。しかしながら、水俣病特措法により救済されなかった人たちについて、環境省と熊本県・鹿児島県は異議申立ができないという態度を取っている。ところが、新潟県では異議申立ができるとしており、水俣病をめぐる行政の対応は別れている。

　こうした中で、さらに水俣病特措法の申請〆切に関連して、国や県は、次の者たちの申請の道を閉ざしたという問題点が指摘されている。

　第1に、濃厚汚染の時期に山間部には行商で汚染魚が運ばれた歴史があり、この発掘調査が遅れていること。

　第2に、熊本や鹿児島で対象地域外に住む人たちの発掘調査である。熊本では天草地域がそうであり、鹿児島でも内陸部がそうである。

　第3に、水俣病が発症したとされる1968年12月までは救済の対象であるが、それ以降生まれたものは対象者とならないということである。もっとも、2011年3月の裁判所での和解では、この制限と第2の制限を受けた者も救済対象としている。今後は水俣病特措法の制限を外す必要があろう。

　第4に、例えば、濃厚汚染地域の津奈木町では、濃厚汚染時期以

降町民の半数が町を出て都会に移り住んでいる。その調査はなされていない。

　ところで、チッソは 2011 年 1 月、水俣病特措法に従い、「JNC 株式会社」を設立し、同年 4 月チッソは JNC に全事業を譲渡した。しかし、2004 年 10 月 15 日、最高裁判所は、感覚障害だけの患者について国と熊本県の賠償責任を認めた。したがって、感覚障害だけの水俣病患者の救済をしない限り、すべての水俣病患者の救済は終わらない。

　さらに、2013 年 4 月 16 日、最高裁判所は、感覚障害だけの患者であっても、行政認定上水俣病であるとして認定する判決を下している。したがって、今後は、感覚障害だけの者であっても、裁判で行政による水俣病患者として認定されるか、民事上の損害賠償を求めることもできることになる。

　そして、2013 年 6 月 20 日、48 人の原告が水俣病患者としての損害賠償を求めて、国・熊本県などを被告に裁判を熊本地裁に提起した。

　政府が、水俣病を公式に確認したのは、1956 年 5 月 1 日である。その日から 57 年経ったが、まだ水俣病をめぐる裁判は続いている。最後の一人の水俣病患者が救済されるまでたたかいは続いていくであろう。

　「公害は被害に始まり被害に終わる」というが、水俣病も未だに解決を見ていないのである。

Appendices

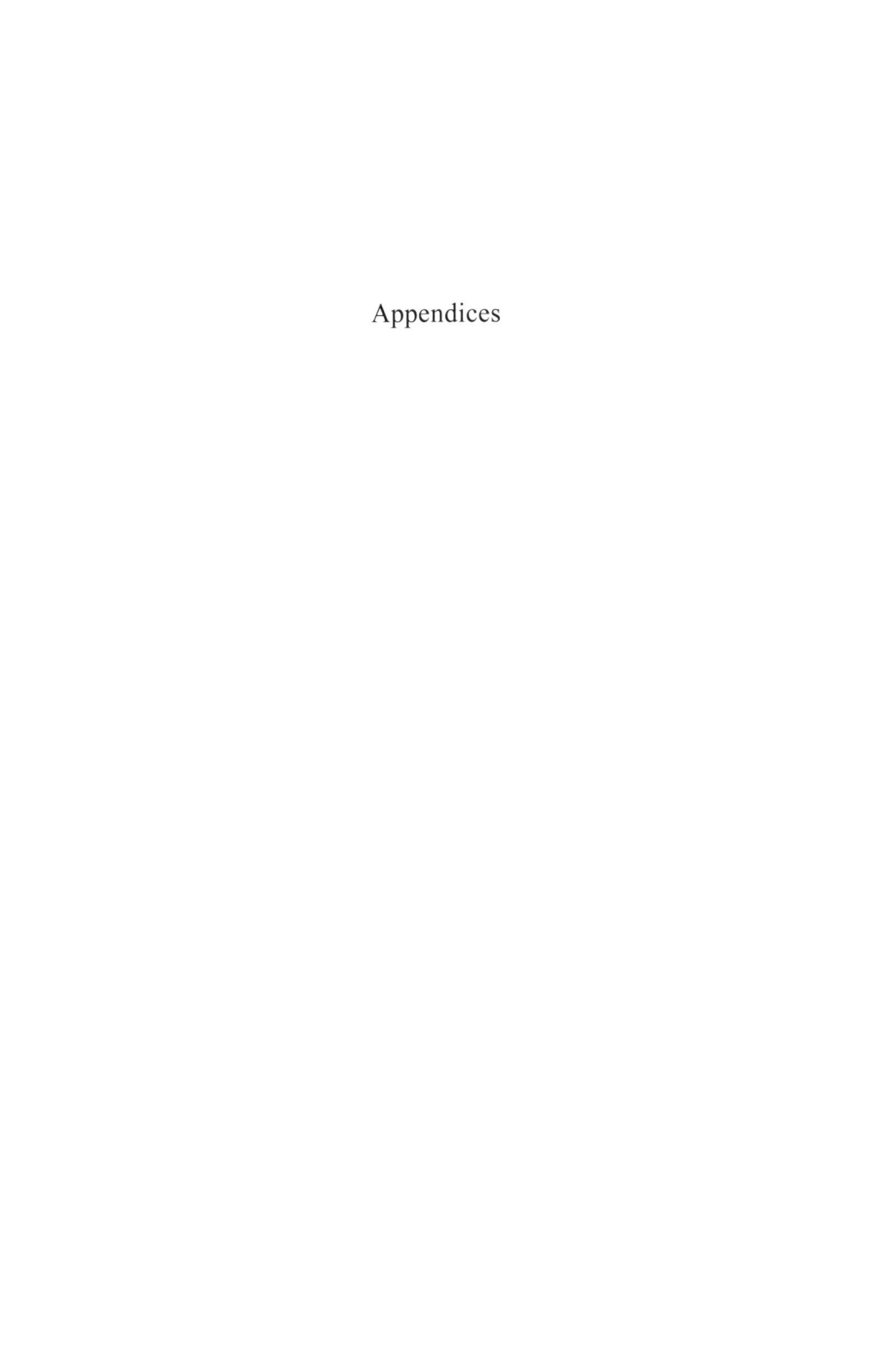

Appendices

1. Timeline of Minamata Disease

Date	Event
January 1906	Shitagau Noguchi builds a power plant in Okuchi, Kagoshima Prefecture, and founds Sogi Electric.
August 1908	Sogi Electric and Nippon Carbide Corporation are merged into Nippon Nitrogen Fertilizer Corporation (Chisso).
March 1932	The Chisso Minamata factory starts producing acetaldehyde using mercury as a catalyst.
June 1955	Cats are exterminated in Modo and Tsukinoura, Minamata City.
May 1956	Hajime Hosokawa, director of the Chisso factory hospital, reports to the Minamata Public Health Center a disease of the central nervous system — suspecting a contagious disease — whose cause is unknown. This turns out to be the official recognition of Minamata disease.
March 1957	The director of the Minamata Public Health Center starts an experiment feeding cats with fish and shellfish from Minamata Bay.
July 1957	The Kumamoto prefectural government considers banning the sale of fish and shellfish from Minamata Bay according to the Food Sanitation Law.
September 1957	But in response to the prefectural government's inquiry about banning the sale of fish and shellfish, the Ministry of Health and Welfare replies, "there is no clear evidence that all fish and shellfish from Minamata Bay are contaminated." As a result, the sale is not banned.
September 1958	Chisso changes the wastewater output route, discharging wastewater into the mouth of the Minamata River instead of Hyakken Harbor.
December 1958	Two laws related to water quality — the Water Quality Control Law and the Factory Effluent Control Law — are enacted. But Chisso is not subject to these laws.

Appendices

October 1959	A mass rally of the Minamata Fishing Cooperative (the First Fishermen's Dispute)
November 1959	A mass rally of the fishing cooperatives in the coastal areas of the Shiranui Sea (the Second Fishermen's Dispute) They demand the suspension of the factory's operation. Rejected their demand, they force their way into the factory and clash with the police force, with more than one hundred injured. (the Chisso Invasion Incident)
December 1959	Chisso and the Patients and Families Mutual Aid Society sign a sympathy money agreement, which does not specify the responsibility and causal relationship.
January 1961	For the Chisso Invasion Incident caused by the fishermen in the coastal areas of the Shiranui Sea, three persons — heads of fishing cooperatives of Tsunagi, Ashikita, and Tanoura — receive a suspended sentence; fifty-two, a fine.
August 1961	Congenial Minamata disease is certified for the first time — the official discovery of congenital Minamata disease.
June 1967	The First Niigata Minamata Disease Lawsuit is filed. The patients of Niigata Minamata disease demand compensation from Showa Denko.
May 1968	The production of acetaldehyde ends in Japan, with Chisso its last manufacturer.
September 1968	The national government recognizes Minamata disease as a pollution-related disease, because it knows that the cause cannot be proved after the half life of methyl mercury in hair passes, with the production of acetaldehyde over.
June 1969	Victims in Kumamoto file a lawsuit demanding compensation from Chisso in the Kumamoto District Court. This is the First Kumamoto Minamata Disease Lawsuit.
September 1971	A decision on the First Niigata Minamata Disease Lawsuit is handed down. The plaintiffs win, but Showa Denko appeals.
January 1973	Certified and as-yet-uncertified patients file a lawsuit demanding compensation from Chisso. The Second Kumamoto Minamata Disease Lawsuit starts.
March 1973	A decision on the First Kumamoto Minamata Disease Lawsuit

Appendices

June 1973	is handed down. The plaintiffs win. In response to the victory of the plaintiffs of Kumamoto Minamata disease, a compensation agreement is also signed in Niigata.
July 1973	Chisso and patients sign a compensation agreement. Chisso pays 16 to 18 million yen per person in compensation to victims' groups recognized by governments.
January 1974	The Kumamoto prefectural government installs dividing nets in Minamata Bay to dispose of sludge containing mercury.
November 1975	Minamata disease patients bring criminal charges against the successive executives of Chisso.
December 1976	In the administrative lawsuit confirming nonfeasance, the victory of plaintiffs is confirmed on the ground that the delay in certification is negligence on the part of governments.
July 1977	It is notified that, "in judging Minamata disease, a combination of multiple symptoms such as motor disturbance, balance disorders, and concentric constriction of the visual field as well as sensory disorders should be used." This is called the 1977 Certification Criteria.
June 1978	A Cabinet meeting approves the Kumamoto prefectural bond to give financial support to Chisso.
March 1979	The president of Chisso and the manager of the Minamata factory are found guilty of professional negligence resulting in death and injury. Later, these sentences are confirmed by the Supreme Court.
August 1985	The Fukuoka High Court hands down its decision on the Second Kumamoto Minamata Disease Lawsuit. It recognizes victims only with sensory disorders as suffering from Minamata disease.
March 1987	The Kumamoto District Court hands down its decision on the First Part of the Third Kumamoto Minamata Disease Lawsuit. It finds the national and prefectural governments as well as Chisso responsible.
February 1988	The Supreme Court hands down its decision on the appellate trial of the Chisso Criminal Trial, dismissing the final appeal.

	The president and factory manager are confirmed guilty. This ruling concludes that they committed injurious assaults or murders on fetuses.
November 1990	The Tokyo District Court issues a recommendation for settlement. But the national government rejects it.
March 1993	The decision on the Second Part of the Third Kumamoto Minamata Disease Lawsuit is handed down. It finds the national and prefectural governments responsible.
December 1995	A Cabinet meeting decides measures concerning Minamata disease, which lead to the 1995 political solution.
May 1996	In the Tokyo High Court, Kumamoto District Court, Osaka High Court, Kyoto District Court, and Fukuoka High Court, settlements are reached with Chisso. Except for the Kansai Lawsuit, all the civil lawsuits concerning Minamata disease are concluded.
October 2004	The Supreme Court hands down its decision on the Minamata Disease Kansai Lawsuit. It finds the national and prefectural governments responsible for compensation, while recognizing sensory disorders as a symptom of Minamata disease.
October 2005	Fifty members of the Association of Minamata Disease Victims "SHIRANUI" file the No-More-Minamata Lawsuit Claiming Government Compensation. The defendants are the national and Kumamoto prefectural governments and Chisso.
April 2006	The number of the plaintiffs of the No-More-Minamata Lawsuit exceeds 1,000. Both Houses adopt the "resolution not to repeat disastrous pollution."
June 2006	The Government Parties' Project Team for Minamata Disease Issues is formed. The additional lawsuit of the No-More-Minamata Lawsuit is filed, bringing the total number of plaintiffs to 1,124.
September 2006	At an international forum concerning environmental damage, where fourteen countries participate, the plaintiff group argues for promulgating the lessons of Minamata disease globally.
November 2006	The number of plaintiffs in the No-More-Minamata Lawsuit reaches 1,159. Chisso seems to contest thoroughly, saying, "we

Appendices

	can't persuade stockholders, employees, and financial institutions of our payments."
January 2007	The Kyushu Federation of Bar Associations warns the national and prefectural governments and Chisso that "neglecting Minamata disease victims is the violation of human rights."
February 2007	The number of the recipients of the new health notebooks exceeds 10,000.
May 2008	Fifty-two years after Minamata disease was officially recognized, the Minister of the Environment, the Kumamoto prefectural governor, and the chair of Chisso attend the Minamata Disease Victims Memorial Service.
June 2009	The Association of Minamata Disease Victims "SHIRANUI" launches a sit-in in front of the office building of the House of Representatives to prevent the enactment of the Law Concerning Special Measures for the Relief of Minamata Disease Victims and the Settlement of Minamata Disease Issues. For this law includes the division of Chisso and the prescription of Minamata disease.
July 2009	The House of Representatives and the House of Councilors pass the Law Concerning Special Measures. The law is enacted.
August 2009	Minamata disease victims' groups and defense teams in Kumamoto, the Kinki Region, and Niigata form the No More Minamata Disease National Liaison Council of Victims and Defense Teams.
September 2009	The Yukio Hatoyama administration is inaugurated. Prime Minister Hatoyama expresses his willingness to accept the opinion presented by the court. Because the Law Concerning Special Measures was enacted, Chisso decides to accept the opinion.
March 2010	In the fifth settlement negotiation in the No-More-Minamata Lawsuit, a "basic agreement" is reached.
May	The Minamata Disease Victims Memorial Service is held in Minamata City. Prime Minister Yukio Hatoyama attends the ceremony as the first prime minister to attend the ceremony and apologizes.

Appendices

June	In one month after the application based on the Law Concerning Special Measures started, a total of 18,458 victims apply in Kumamoto and Kagoshima Prefectures.
September	The number of applicants for relief based on the law amounts to 34,028 by August.
January 2011	Chisso is divided according to the law, establishing a company, "JNC Inc."
March 2011	A settlement is reached in the No-More-Minamata Niigata Lawsuit for the Relief of All Victims involving 173 plaintiffs. The number of applicants based on the law exceeds 40,000. The Great East Japan Earthquake occurs, causing an accident at the Fukushima Daiichi Nuclear Power Plant. Settlements are reached in the No-More-Minamata Tokyo (194 plaintiffs), Kumamoto (2,492 plaintiffs), and Osaka Lawsuits (306 plaintiffs).
April 2011	Chisso transfers all its businesses to JNC Inc.
July 2012	The number of applicants based on the law amounts to about 70,000.

Appendices

2. Population Change in Minamata City

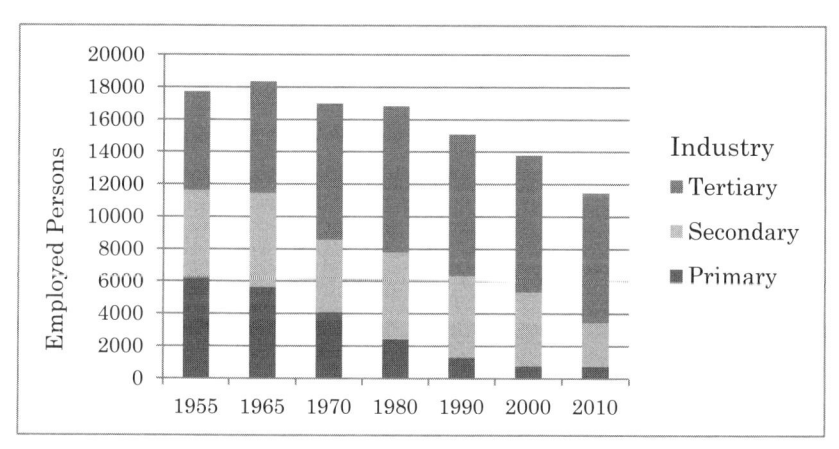

Figure 4. Employed persons by industry

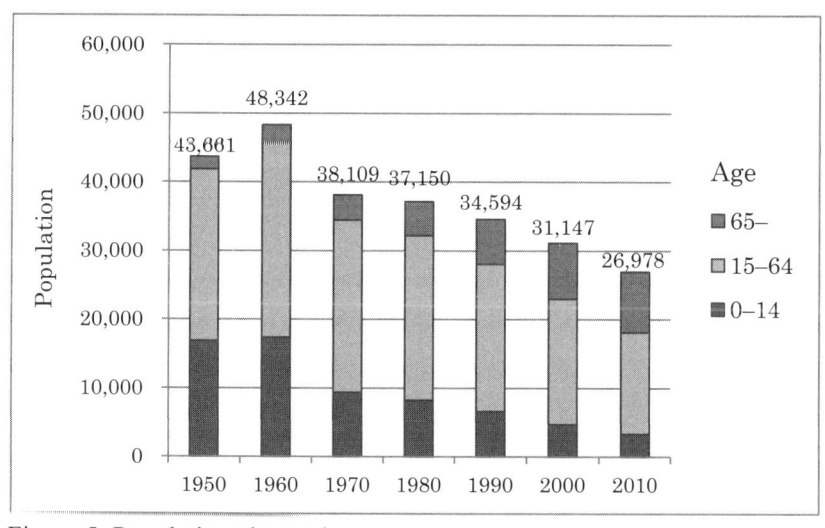

Figure 5. Population change by age group

3. Japanese–English Glossary for Minamata disease issues

50音	Japanese	English
あ	アミン中毒説	the Amino poisoning theory
か	桂島	Katsura Island
か	関西訴訟	the Kansai Lawsuit
か	患者・家庭互助会	the Patients and Families Mutual Aid Society
き	奇病	the strange disease
き	救済対象者	relief recipients
き	共通診断書	the uniform medical certificate
ぎ	行政の根幹論	the theory of the foundation of governance
く	熊本水俣病第一次訴訟	the First Kumamoto Minamata Disease Lawsuit
こ	厚生省食品衛生調査会水俣食中毒部会	the Minamata Food Poisoning Special Committee of the Ministry of Health and Welfare's Food Sanitation Investigation Council
さ	サイクレーター	the Cyclator
し	司法救済制度	a judicial relief scheme
し	昭和52年判断条件	the 1977 Certification Criteria
し	不知火海	the Shiranui Sea
し	四肢末梢優位の表在感覚障害	superficial sensory disorders in the distal portion of all four extremities
じ	重金属説	the heavy metal poisoning theory
せ	政府解決案	the draft of the Final Solution Scheme
ぜ	全国公害被害者総行動	the Nationwide General Action of Pollution Victims
ぜ	全日本民医連	the Japan Federation of Democratic Medical Institutions
そ	総合対策医療事業	the comprehensive medical care project
だ	大検診	the Mass Medical Examinations
ち	チッソ	Chisso Corporation (Chisso)
ち	チッソ付属病院	the Chisso factory hospital

ち	チッソ水俣工場	the Chisso Minamata factory
に	日本化学工業会	the Japan Chemical Industry Association
に	日本窒素株式会社	Nippon Nitrogen Fertilizer Corporation
に	認定審査会	the certification committee
の	ノーモア・ミナマタ国家賠償等訴訟	the No-More-Minamata Lawsuit Claiming Government Compensation
の	ノーモア・ミナマタ水俣病被害者・弁護団全国連絡会議（全国連）	the No More Minamata Disease National Liaison Council of Victims and Defense Teams (the No More Council)
ひ	樋島	Hino Island
ひ	百間排水路	the Hyakken Waterway
み	水俣川	Minamata River
み	水俣漁協	the Minamata Fishing Cooperative
み	水俣湾	Minamata Bay
み	未認定患者	as-yet-uncertified patients
み	見舞金契約	a sympathy money agreement
み	水俣病犠牲者慰霊式	the Minamata Disease Victims Memorial Service
み	水俣病県民会議医師団	the team of medical doctors of the Minamata Disease Citizens' Council
み	水俣病闘争支援熊本県連絡会議	the Kumamoto Prefecture Liaison Council to Support Minamata Disease Battles
み	水俣病被害者の救済及び水俣病問題の解決に関する特別措置法	the Law Concerning Special Measures for the Relief of Minamata Disease Victims and the Settlement of Minamata Disease Issues
み	水俣病不知火患者会	the Association of Minamata Disease Victims "SHIRANUI" (Association "SHIRANUI")
み	水俣病問題懇談会	the Council on Minamata Disease Issues
み	水俣病問題与党プロジェクトチーム	the Government Parties' Project Team for Minamata Disease Issues
み	民主党水俣病対策作業チーム	the Democratic Party's Minamata Disease Working Team
ゆ	有機水銀説	the organic mercury theory

Index

1977 Certification Criteria 29, 48
1995 political solution 32, 33, 35, 50, 53
2004 Supreme Court decision 33, 35, 38, 50, 53, 65, 67
acetaldehyde 19, 21, 25, 26, 28, 51
Amino poisoning theory 24
Association "SHIRANUI" 34, 37, 39, 40, 42, 57, 66
as-yet-uncertified patients 29
castle town 13, 19, 28
cat experiment 24, 26
Chisso Minamata factory 24, 25, 26
Environment Agency 30
extinctive prescription 49, 50, 52, 61, 70
Factory Effluent Control Law 25
First Kumamoto Minamata Disease Lawsuit 27, 28, 50
Food Sanitation Law 25
Government Parties' Project Team for Minamata Disease Issues 43, 57
Hajime Hosokawa 21
heavy metal poisoning theory 25
Hyakken Waterway 26
Kagoshima Prefecture 19, 42, 71
Kansai Lawsuit 32, 33, 35, 50, 53, 65, 67
Kumamoto Prefecture 17, 19, 53, 63, 71
Kumamoto University 21, 24, 27
Law Concerning Special Measures 44, 56, 57, 58, 59, 61, 67, 69, 70, 71
Masazumi Harada 42, 45, 62
Masazumi Yoshii 64
Mass Medical Examinations 40, 42, 43, 52
methyl mercury 17, 19, 25, 33, 46, 47, 51, 66, 69

Index

Minamata Caravan	53
Minamata City	13, 17, 62, 63
Minamata Public Health Center	21
Ministry of the Environment	34, 66, 71
Motoo Fujiki	49, 51
Niigata Minamata disease	17
organic mercury	11, 17, 24, 25, 27
Science and Technology Agency	26
Second Kumamoto Minamata Disease Lawsuit	29
Shigeru Takaoka	46, 47, 51, 53, 61, 68
Showa Denko	12, 17
sympathy money agreement	26, 29
term of exclusion	49, 50, 51, 52, 61, 69
Ministry of Health and Welfare	24, 25
theory of the foundation of governance	38, 68
Third Kumamoto Minamata Disease Lawsuit	30, 37, 51
third-party committee	63, 64, 68
uniform medical certificate	45, 46, 47, 48, 49, 68
Water Quality Control Law	25

水俣病不知火患者会、ノーモア・ミナマタ国賠等訴訟弁護団、
ノーモア・ミナマタ編集委員会　編
監訳　鳥飼香代子、土肥勲嗣

英語版・日本語版　ノーモア・ミナマタ──司法による解決のみち
Court Battles over a Pollution-Related Disease　*The Case of Minamata Disease*

2013年10月1日　初版第1刷発行

編著 ──── 水俣病不知火患者会、ノーモア・ミナマタ国賠等訴訟弁護団、
　　　　　　ノーモア・ミナマタ編集委員会
発行者 ──── 平田　勝
発行 ──── 花伝社
発売 ──── 共栄書房
〒101-0065　東京都千代田区西神田2-5-11出版輸送ビル2F
電話　　　03-3263-3813
FAX　　　03-3239-8272
E-mail　　kadensha@muf.biglobe.ne.jp
URL　　　http://kadensha.net
振替　　　00140-6-59661
装幀 ──── 佐々木正見
印刷・製本 ─ シナノ印刷株式会社

ⓒ2013 水俣病不知火患者会、ノーモア・ミナマタ国賠等訴訟弁護団、ノーモア・ミナマタ編集委員会
ISBN978-4-7634-0678-1 C0036

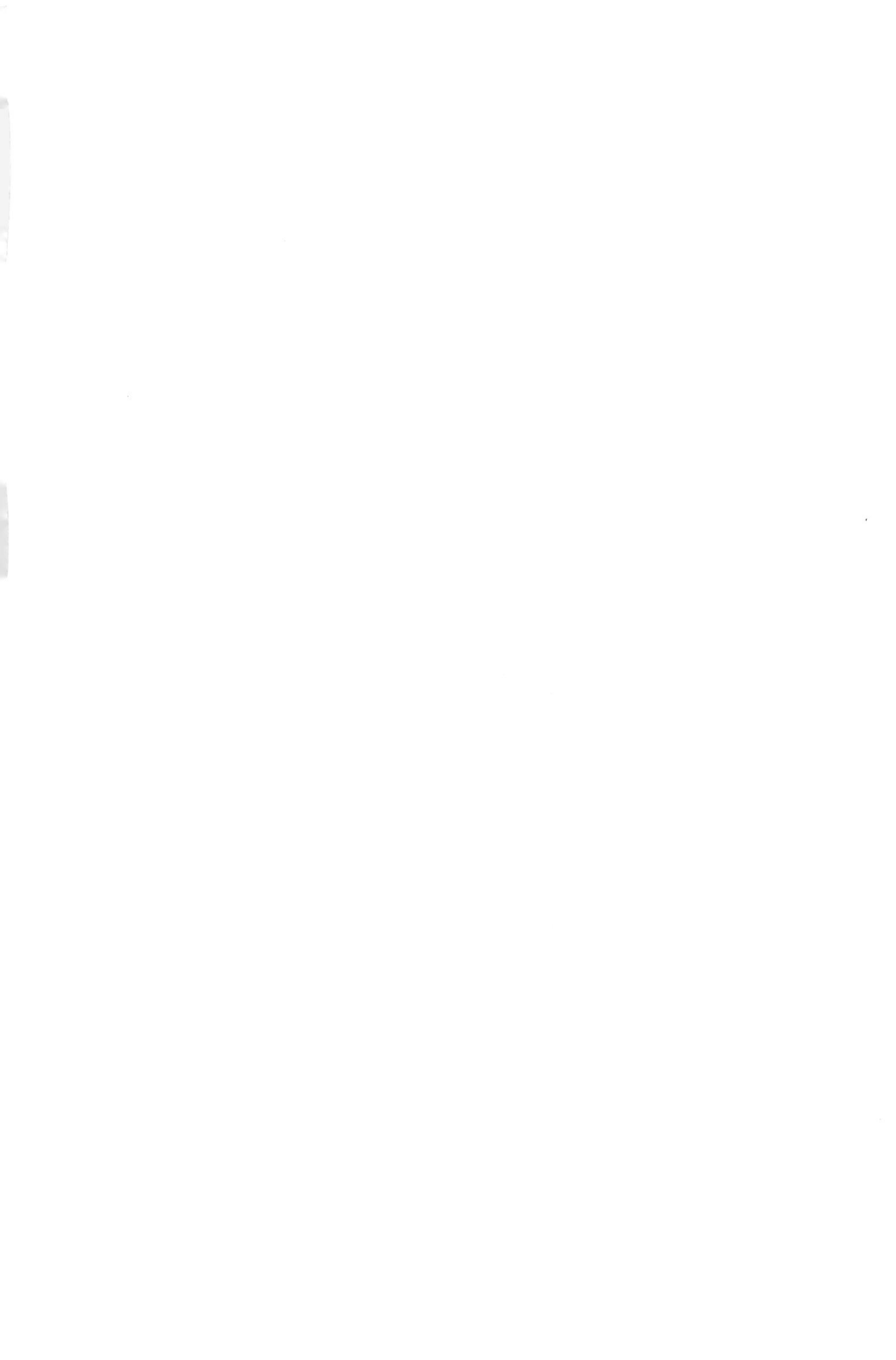